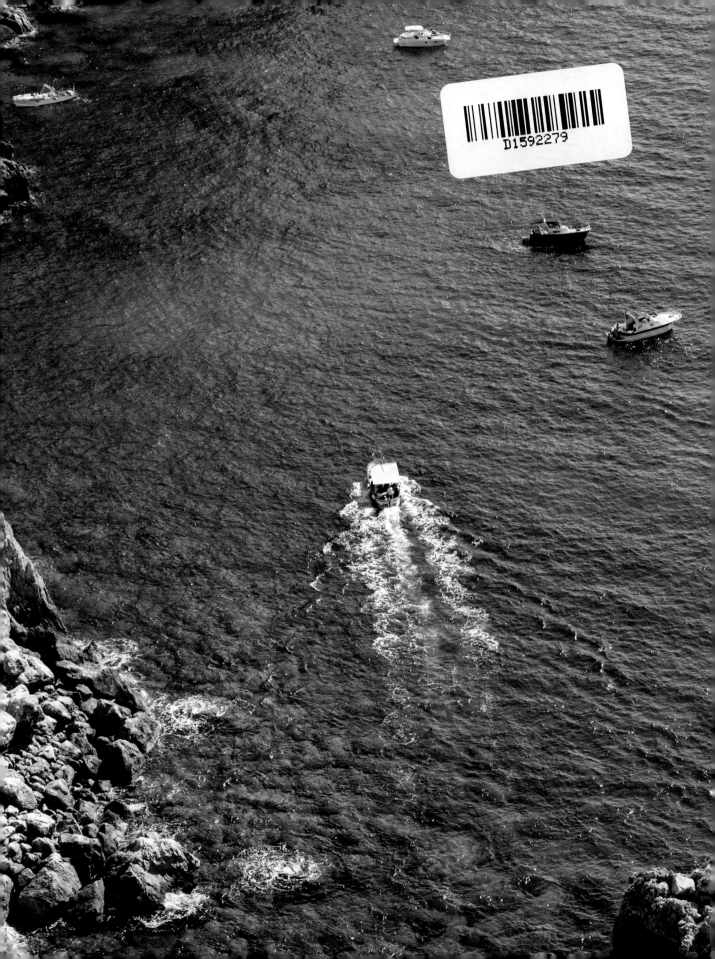

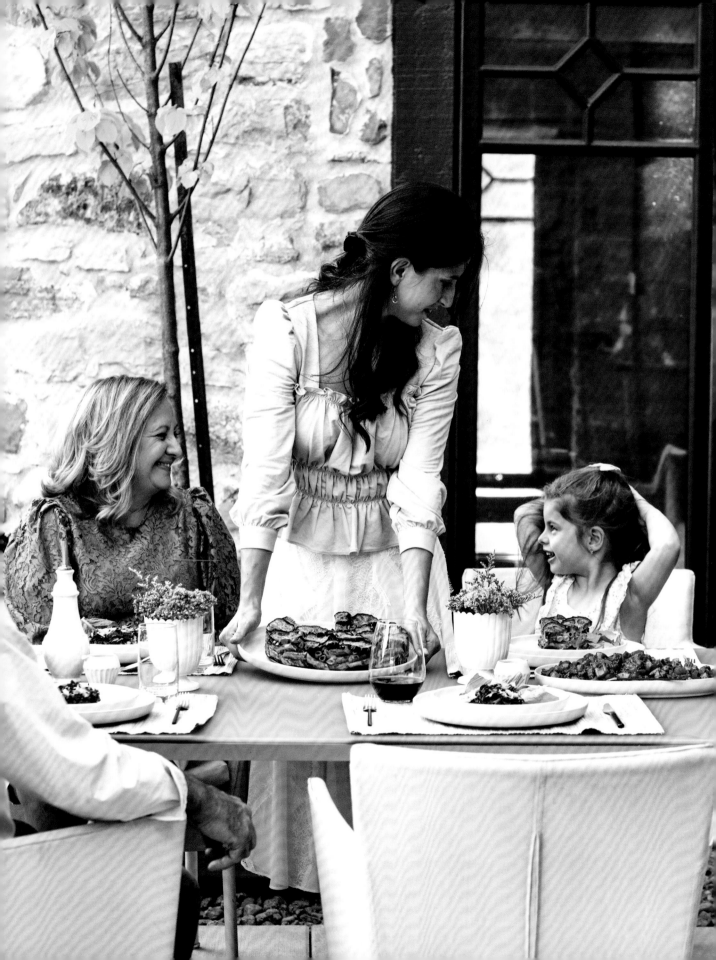

Everyday Mediterranean

A Complete Guide to the Mediterranean Diet

with 90+ Simple, Nourishing Recipes

~

Vanessa Perrone, MS, RD

appetite
by RANDOM HOUSE

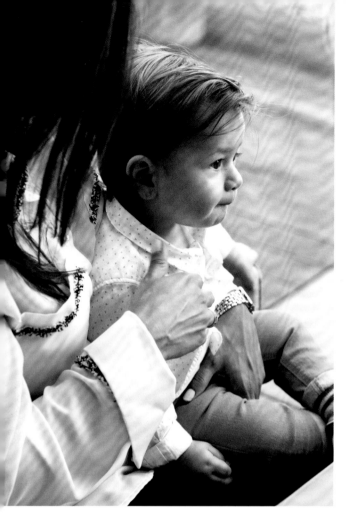

Appetite by Random House® and colophon are registered trademarks of Penguin Random House LLC.

Library and Archives Canada Cataloguing in Publication is available upon request.

ISBN: 978-0-525-61185-1
eBook ISBN: 978-0-525-61186-8

Book design: Lisa Jager
Interior photography: Ariel Tarr

Author note: The content of this book is for education purposes only and is not meant to replace medical advice. For recommendations that meet your specific health needs, contact your physician, registered dietitian, or other healthcare professional.

Printed in China

Published in Canada by Appetite by Random House®, a division of Penguin Random House Canada Limited.

www.penguinrandomhouse.ca

10 9 8 7 6 5 4 3 2 1

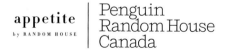

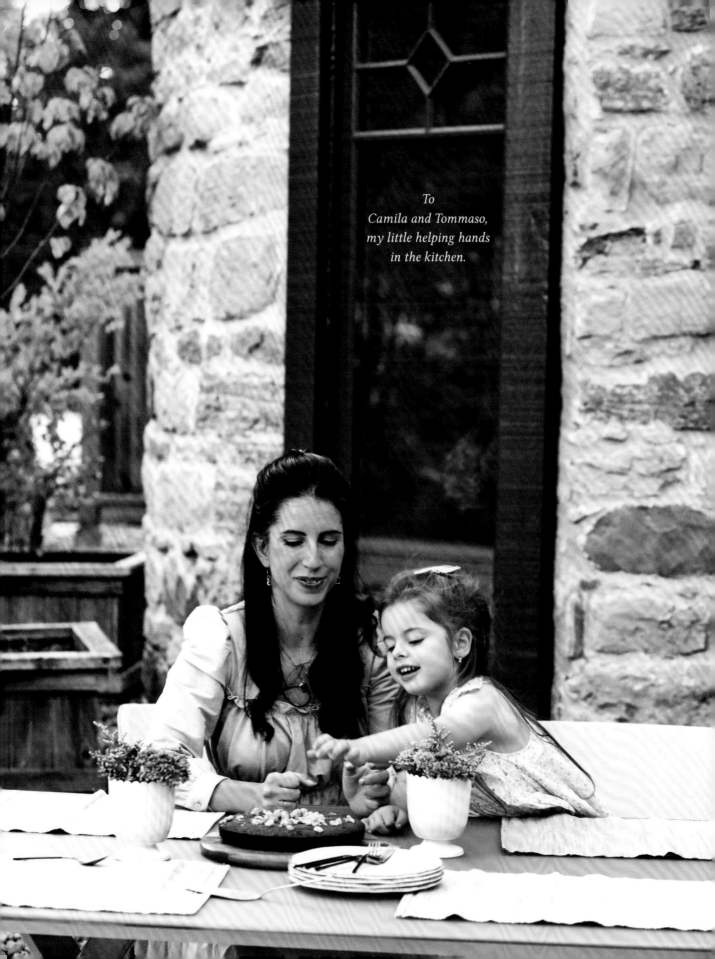

To
*Camila and Tommaso,
my little helping hands
in the kitchen.*

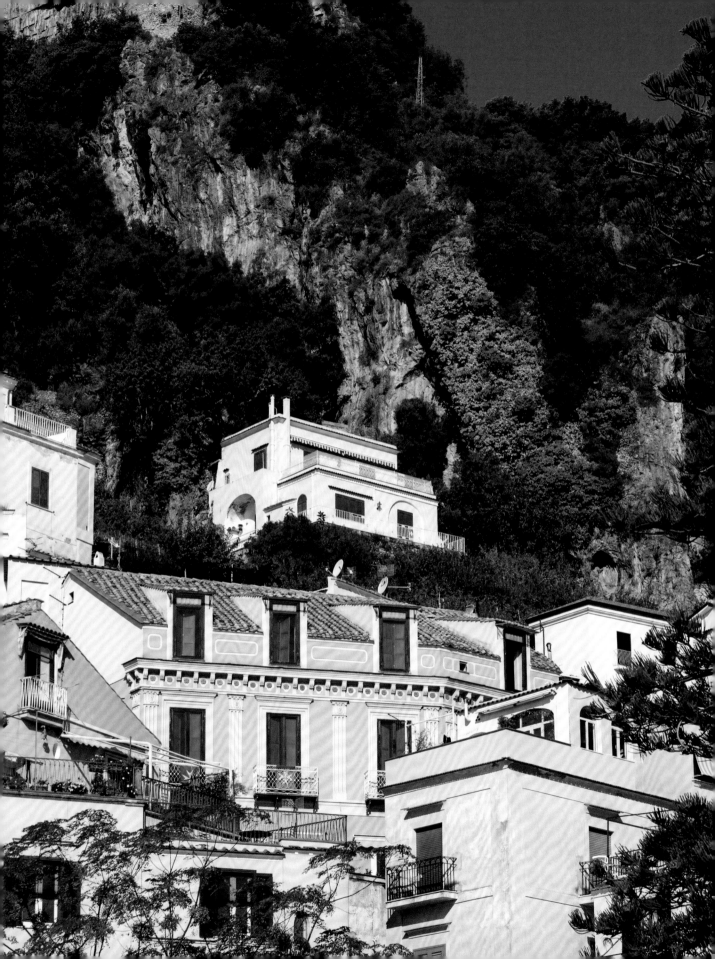

Contents

Meat

Sunday Gathering

Sweets and Desserts

Basics

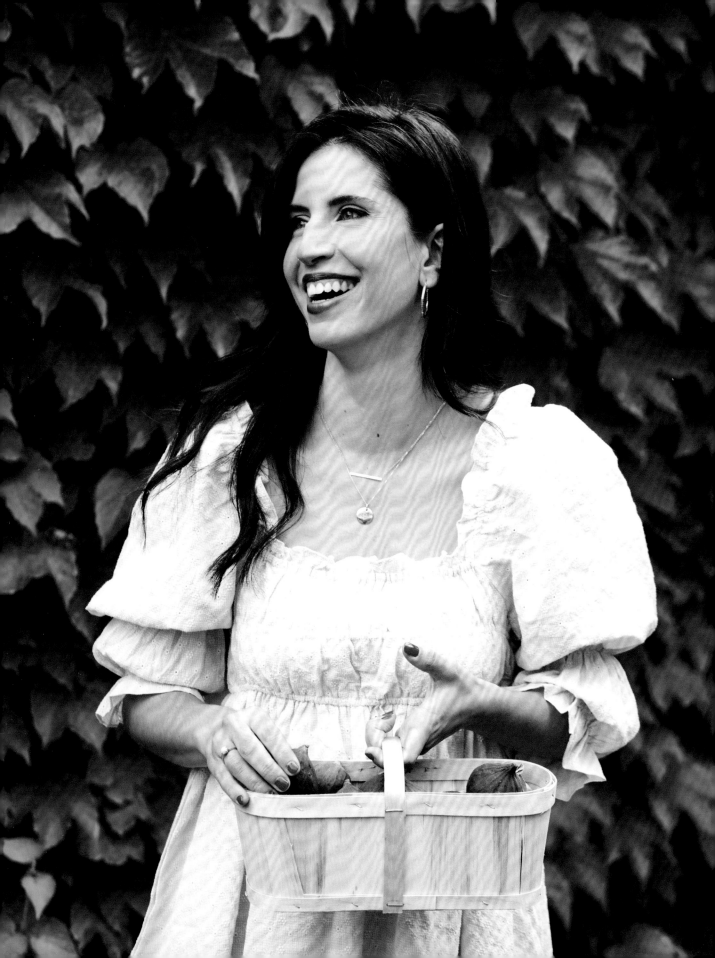

Introduction

There is no *best* diet.

Considering the title of this book, this statement may come as a surprise. But while there is no best diet per se, there is a best way to eat for *you*. Your aim should be to find an eating pattern that will nourish your body but still feed your soul and please your taste buds—a way of eating that is easy and delicious, and avoids compromise.

As it turns out, the Mediterranean diet is not an eating pattern that I, nor anyone else, created. As we'll discuss, it isn't a diet at all. It represents the traditional eating pattern of real individuals who went about their lifestyle as best they knew how and happened to become one of history's healthiest populations. The Mediterranean diet is characterized by plant-centric meals, seasonality, daily physical activity, and regular sharing of meals. So, although the Mediterranean diet is traditional, its principles are flexible and still translate to today. I learned of the benefits of the Mediterranean diet in university and now use it as a tool in my practice to prevent and treat chronic diseases. But I mostly learned the principles of a Mediterranean diet at home.

When you're born into an Italian family, you inherit an almost innate passion for food that feels nothing short of winning a food culture lottery. Growing up, I witnessed culinary traditions passing down generations; some of my fondest memories were formed in the kitchen, and I felt my deepest emotions at the dinner table. This upbringing fanned the initial spark, and my passion for food began to grow. Food remains the center of my universe, as I wear the hat of both mom and dietitian. In my professional world, I use food as a tool to nourish, prevent, and heal. At home, food is synonymous with tradition, culture, and celebration, all of which are essential to my healthy-living prescription.

This crossover of personal and professional life has inspired me to share the magic of the Mediterranean eating pattern with you. So, while there is no *best* diet, my mission in sharing with you the principles of the Mediterranean diet is to inspire you to adopt a nutritious, delicious way of eating that fits into your everyday without compromise.

Sadly, it's become too easy to lose touch with our food cultures. Diet culture is stronger than ever before, and this dangerous trade-off puts relationships with food, body image, and health at risk. Add this to work-life balance struggles and you may wonder if it is possible to eat well and feel well while still finding joy in eating.

Fortunately, there *is* a way to strike that delicate balance that is compatible with our modern lives. And I'm here to tell you how. Welcome to *Everyday Mediterranean*, a guide to eating well and living well according to the traditional Mediterranean diet. The Mediterranean diet has stood the test of time as one of the healthiest eating patterns ever studied, with decades (and counting) of research supporting its benefits. The pattern and its principles have become a gold standard for lifelong health. In this book, you will learn the fundamental principles of the Mediterranean diet—and how to apply them to your life—through tips and recipes inspired by my heritage and favorite Mediterranean ingredients. There's a little something for everyone—from olive oil granola to spinach falafel to baklava-style apple strudel and figgy energy bites.

I am delighted to bring tradition, modern inspiration, and flavor to your daily table so that you too can make every day Mediterranean.

Buon appetito,
Vanessa

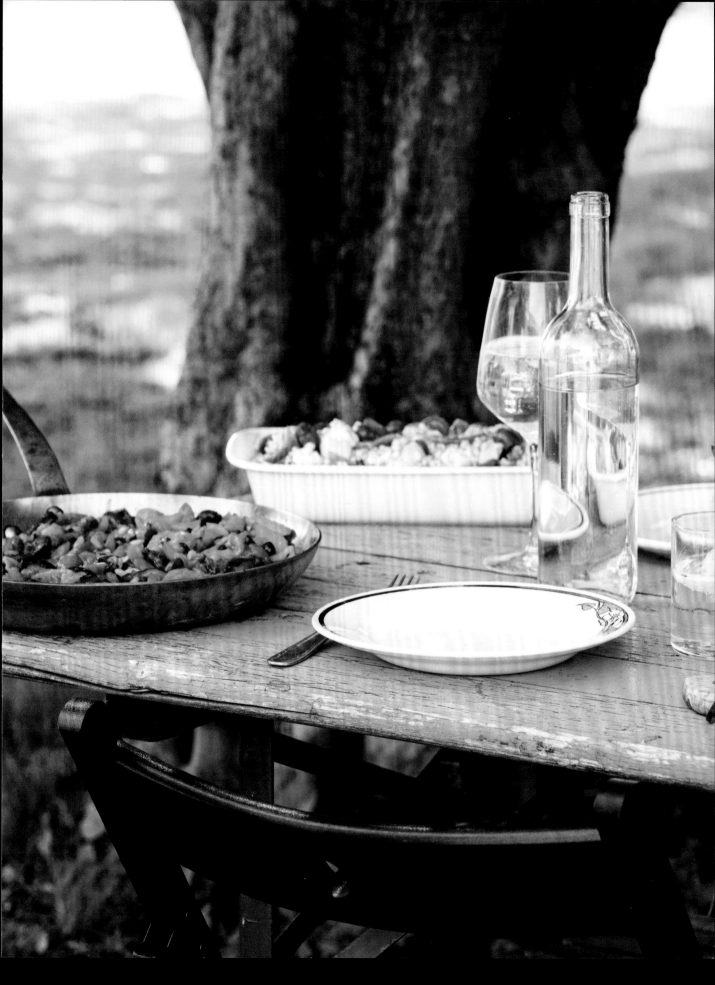

Living the Mediterranean Way

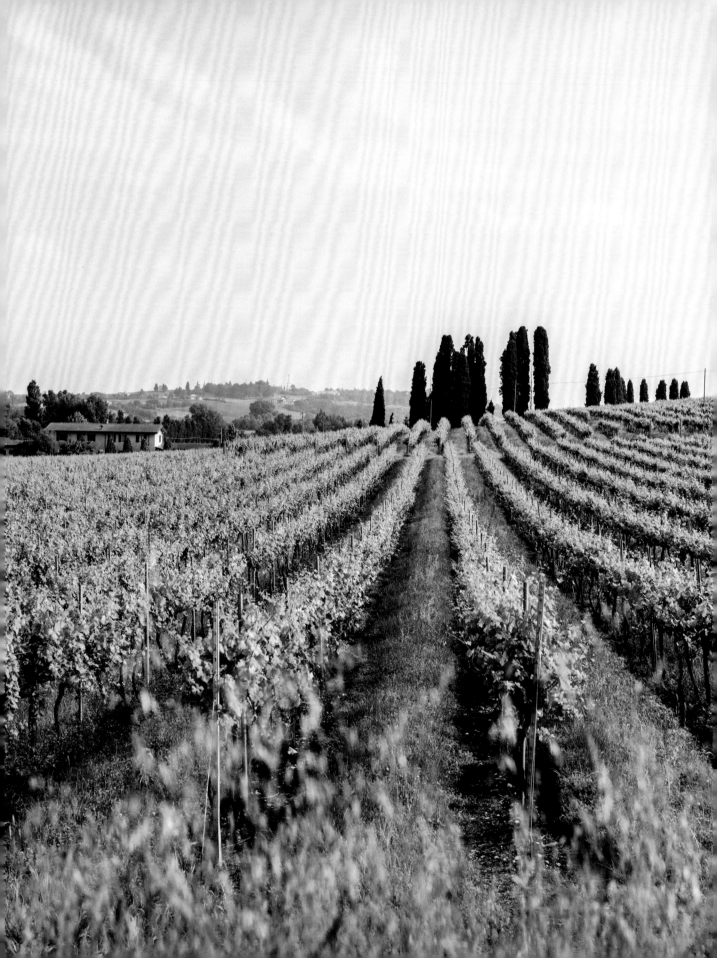

What Is the Mediterranean Diet?

A warm breeze, the sun on your skin, pastel-colored villas propped against a clear blue sky and a glistening sea . . . these are the images that come to mind when we hear the word "Mediterranean." "Mediterranean *diet*," however, conjures much more than a picturesque landscape. Imagine a long table set outdoors, covered with platters of traditional dishes made with seasonal ingredients. Around the table sits a family who will share in these meals, connect, and celebrate, as they do every week. This scene captures the essence of the Mediterranean diet and the key message of this chapter: that the Mediterranean diet is more than just a way of *eating*. It is a way of *living* that we can adapt wherever we are.

A Traditional Eating Pattern

The Mediterranean diet is a traditional eating pattern characterized by an abundance of vegetables and fruit; a high consumption of pulses, whole grains, and nuts; and a high intake of extra virgin olive oil. There is frequent consumption of fish and seafood; moderate consumption of animal protein, such as poultry, eggs, and dairy; regular but moderate consumption of red wine; and low consumption of red meat and sweets, which are eaten only in small amounts.

The Discovery

More than 50 years ago on the Mediterranean coast, inhabitants of Crete and Southern Italy unexpectedly displayed some of the lowest rates of chronic disease in the world, with adult life expectancy among the highest

7

despite their poor living conditions. Intrigued, researchers turned to their plates to investigate their eating habits and understand how these individuals had come to be some of the healthiest on earth. When they discovered their nutritionally sound eating habits, they made the connection between their diet and health, which led to the coining of the term "Mediterranean diet," reflecting the eating pattern of those living in olive-growing regions of the Mediterranean in the early 1960s.

A Flexible Model

There is no one pure Mediterranean diet, since each region has its own culinary and cultural traditions; as such, there's no one strict definition of it. However, key principles of this healthful pattern stood out across Mediterranean populations and were combined to form the model we know today.

DIETARY TRAITS OF THE MEDITERRANEAN DIET

- Few processed foods
- A high intake and variety of vegetables
- Whole grains and pulses as the base of meals
- Fresh fruit daily, often for dessert
- Water or herbal teas several times a day
- Fresh herbs and spices daily

- Nuts, seeds, and olives regularly
- Extra virgin olive oil daily, as the main fat
- Fish regularly
- Animal protein in moderation
- Regular, but moderate, red wine with meals
- Red meat and sweets, occasionally

THE RESULTING NUTRITIONAL CHARACTERISTICS OF THE MEDITERRANEAN DIET

- Low in saturated fat
- Free of trans fats
- Low in added sugar
- Rich in monounsaturated and poly-unsaturated fats
- High in fiber
- Rich in vitamins and minerals

- High plant:animal fat ratio
- High monounsaturated:saturated fat ratio
- Rich in phenolic compounds with antioxidant and anti-inflammatory activity
- Rich in complex carbohydrates

A Way of Life

As I say, the Mediterranean diet is not a diet; it's a lifestyle. You have to look beyond the ingredients on the plate to the lifestyle habits of the Mediterranean people that have played an important part in what makes this way of life so beneficial.

An Enjoyable Model

In discussions of the Mediterranean diet, the word "diet" is a bit of a misnomer. Unlike restrictive nutrition-based diets of today, the Mediterranean diet isn't governed by restrictions or by "good" and "bad" foods. Instead, the Mediterranean diet represents an entire collection of lifestyle practices that include cooking, physical activity, conviviality, and regular sharing of meals. This 360-degree approach is one reason the Mediterranean diet is considered as a sustainable, long-term model. You aren't "on a diet" but, rather, adopting lifelong practices that affect physical, emotional, and social health, and which you can enjoy and ultimately stick with.

THE MEDITERRANEAN LIFESTYLE MEANS . . .

- Daily physical activity
- Meals eaten as a family
- Simple cooking, every day
- Honoring local food products
- Focusing on seasonal or self-harvested produce, when possible

- Eating slowly, and savoring food
- Taking care of your ingredients, without waste
- Cooking mindfully, without rushing

A Humble Cuisine

The Mediterranean diet is the result of a necessary frugality—so much so that it was initially referred to as "the poor man's diet." The fact that it resulted in such beneficial health effects was, as mentioned, what first caught the interest of researchers.

The Poor Man Paradox

After World War II, rural Mediterranean communities faced much hardship. Food items such as meat, sugar, and certain dairy products were either too expensive or too hard to come by to regularly feature in daily cooking.

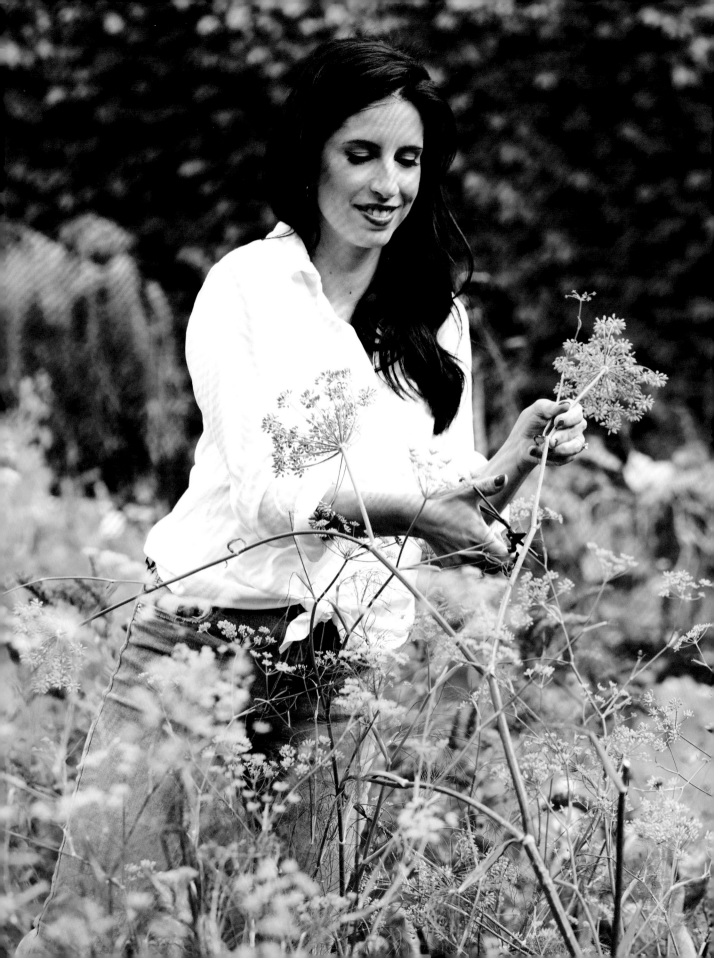

Lacking the means to treat themselves to luxury items, locals relied on more accessible ingredients, like freshly harvested vegetables, fruit, grains, and pulses. The result? Their diet became rich in:

- Pulses
- Whole grains
- Olives and olive oil
- Fresh herbs, wild field greens, and herbal teas
- Fresh fruits and garden vegetables
- Local fish and seafood
- Red wine

So while frugality gave birth to a poor man's diet, the result was, in fact, quite rich in nutrition.

Eating Well, Frugally

Does the Mediterranean diet still fit the bill as a poor man's diet? Not quite. With the rising cost of food, I'm sure "frugal" isn't the word that comes to mind when the cashier rings up your grocery bill. It undoubtedly costs more to eat a nutritious diet today than it once did. That said, there is still much you can do to optimize your food budget and get the most bang for your bite, including:

- **Purchase bulk quantities of foods and split them among family members**: In my family, we do this with things like pricier cheeses (such as Parmigiano Reggiano and Romano), opting for big blocks and then splitting them among my parents, sister, and me. This brings down the cost and allows us all to get a nice variety.
- **Embrace frozen foods**: Just as nutritious as fresh, frozen options often cost less. Explore ingredients like broad beans, kale, spinach, artichoke hearts, and more.
- **Lean in to pulses**: Canned or dried, beans, chickpeas (technically, a type of bean), and lentils are rich in protein and fiber, making them affordable alternatives to meat.
- **Reduce your meat consumption**: To offset the price of foods such as olive oil, nuts, and produce, reduce meat consumption by incorporating plant-based options such as beans and lentils.
- **Treat fresh ingredients with care**: Mindfully storing your fresh ingredients, especially produce, as soon as you return from the grocery store will keep them fresher longer and prevent waste.

- **Plan ahead:** Reducing waste may not reduce the price of your grocery bill, but you make the most of your money. Menu planning and buying just the ingredients you need are key.

- **Grow what you can:** Season and space permitting, growing your own produce is not only cost-effective but helps cultivate a deeper connection with food.

- **Follow the seasons:** For more economical and flavorful options, stock up on seasonal produce. Micronutrient and polyphenol content is also at its peak then. Turn an abundance of seasonal produce into preserves, tomato sauce, or caponata—or simply blanch and freeze for use later in the year. This may involve investing time into transforming the produce, but it will be worth the extra mile.

- **Buy local:** No need to eat Mediterranean ingredients in order to follow a Mediterranean eating pattern. Choosing a local apple rather than an imported pomegranate meets the same principle, but costs less.

- **Use the whole food:** Use vegetable scraps to make broth, Parmigiano Reggiano rind in soup to add flavor, and leftover bread for breadcrumbs, for example. Leave nothing behind.

- **Think outside the box:** Escarole, dandelion greens, canned sardines, and cabbage—these lesser-used ingredients are highly nutritious and affordable too.

- **Embrace dried products:** Dried lentils, dried fruit, dried mushrooms, sun-dried tomatoes, and dried olives are examples of ingredients that can make or enhance a meal.

- **Plant a year-round herb garden:** A windowsill herb garden is a more economical option than store-bought packaged options.

Healthy and Wealthy?

Italian researchers set out to determine how a Mediterranean diet affected various socioeconomic groups, and found that its heart-protective effects were confined to higher earners. Unlike the rural Mediterranean of the 1960s, the rising cost of food, specifically nutrient-dense food, has created inequities in nutrient intake, making it harder to stick to a traditional Mediterranean diet, especially among those who are young or have a lower socioeconomic status. These disparities are unfair and need the attention of government and policy makers so that fresh and nutritious food can stay accessible to us all.

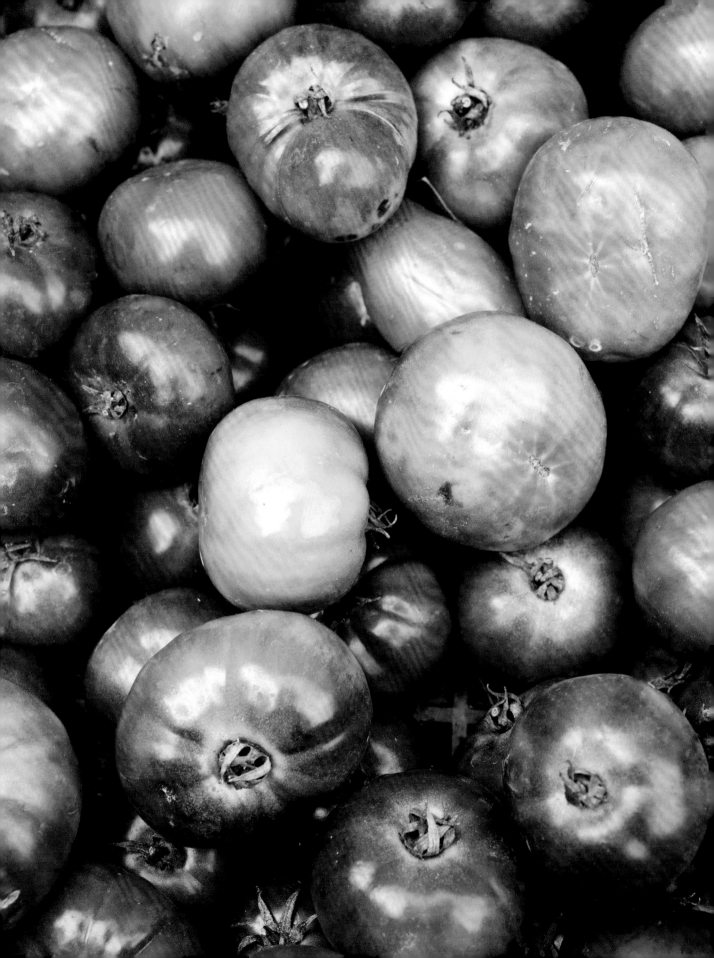

A Diet You Can Stick With

The Mediterranean diet and its benefits have long been touted. Several studies across various fields have shown advantages ranging from longevity to protection against chronic disease and more. But most importantly? The diet also happens to be one of the most accessible patterns we could follow.

A Lifelong Pattern

As a dietitian, I like to tell patients "If you can't give it five years, don't give it five minutes" when they ask me about diets and trends. That's because an important yet often overlooked factor in nutrition is the sustainability of any diet. A diet may be among the healthiest, but you will reap the benefits only if you stick to it. When comparing people's levels of adherence to the Mediterranean diet with that of other popular diets, it always comes out on top. Why? Because it is not defined by strict rules, labels, or deprivation. Instead, it's made of attractive lifestyle habits such as cooking, meal sharing, and daily movement. There also aren't any off-limit foods; rather, the Mediterranean diet uses principles to guide the proportions certain foods should have in your diet (we'll look at this in more detail in the next chapter). For example, animal products and sugar aren't banned; they simply aren't to be consumed on a daily basis like plant-based products are. Finally, and most importantly, the food proposed for a Mediterranean diet is simple and absolutely delicious, both essential factors for anyone considering the lifestyle change. It all makes for a long-term, enjoyable approach that you won't feel like quitting.

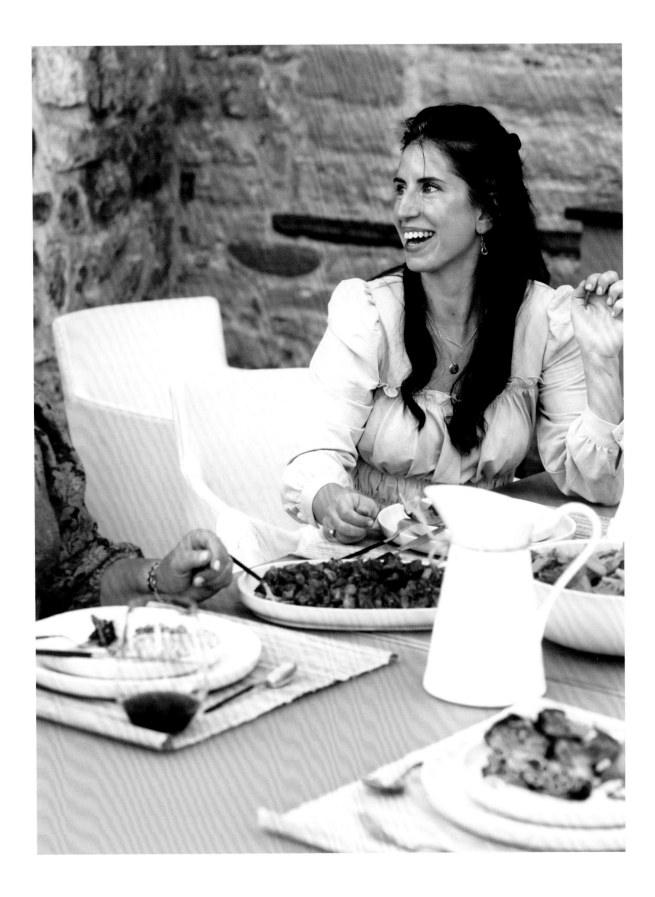

The Principles

Since its discovery, scientists have been dissecting the Mediterranean diet to isolate the source of its benefits. Is it a specific food? Is it a nutrient? If there's one takeaway from the research, it is that the whole is more than the sum of its parts. The synergistic effect of food and lifestyle components is responsible for the Mediterranean diet's benefits. This chapter explores the various principles that make up this pattern.

The Mediterranean Pyramid

The evidence that the Mediterranean diet improves multiple health outcomes is undeniably strong (see more on this in "The Benefits," page 42). But what exactly does the Mediterranean diet look like? On page 18 is a pyramid model, based on the models that have been developed over the years to help answer this question.

The first thing you will notice about the Mediterranean Diet Pyramid is its pattern reflects, above all, a lifestyle, with community as the foundational pillar. Physical activity, cooking, sharing meals, preserving food traditions, and eating with the seasons are habits at the core of this way of life. The pyramid model also highlights that the Mediterranean diet is a plant-forward eating pattern, with vegetables, fruit, whole grains, pulses, nuts, seeds, and extra virgin olive oil consumed on a regular basis. It isn't, however, free of animal protein—you will see fish, dairy, eggs, and poultry present, on a daily to weekly basis. Finally, at the top of the pyramid are red meat and sweets— again, still included, but present only on occasion (weekly to monthly).

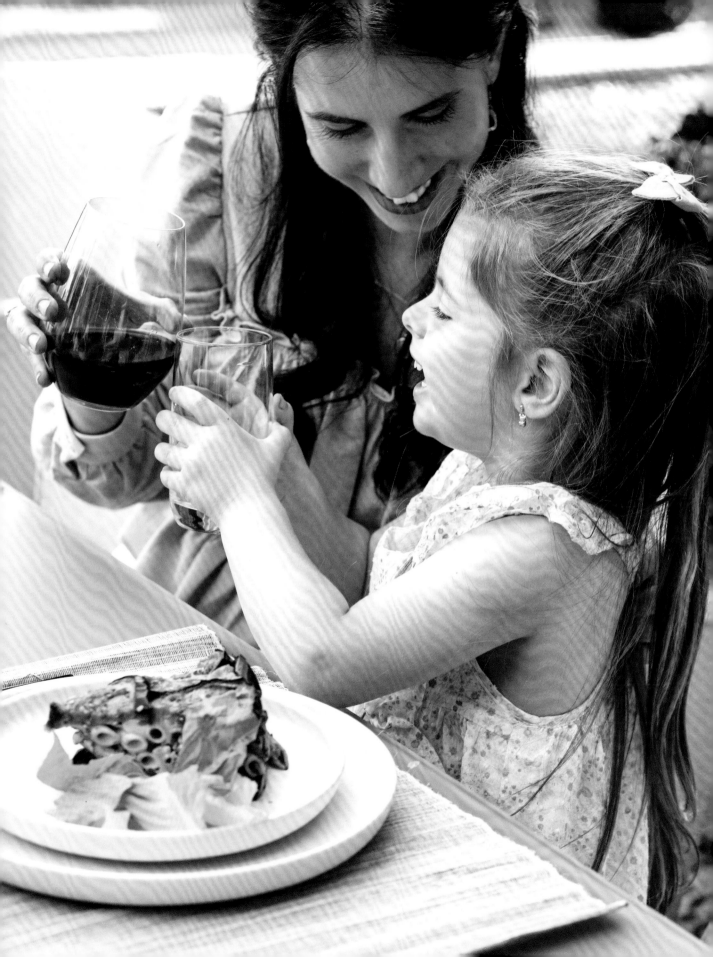

The Mediterranean Diet Pyramid

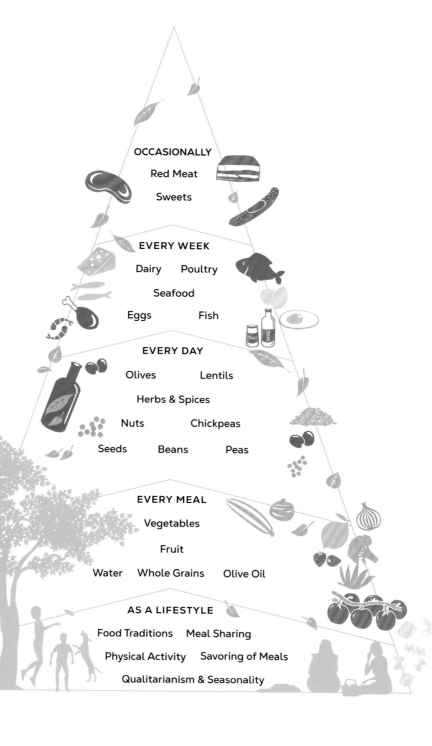

OCCASIONALLY

Red Meat

Sweets

EVERY WEEK

Dairy   Poultry

Seafood

Eggs   Fish

EVERY DAY

Olives   Lentils

Herbs & Spices

Nuts   Chickpeas

Seeds   Beans   Peas

EVERY MEAL

Vegetables

Fruit

Water   Whole Grains   Olive Oil

AS A LIFESTYLE

Food Traditions   Meal Sharing

Physical Activity   Savoring of Meals

Qualitarianism & Seasonality

The Principles of the Mediterranean Diet

Considering what we see in the Mediterranean Diet Pyramid, here are my 10 principles for adopting a Mediterranean lifestyle:

1. Focus on food traditions.
2. Share meals with loved ones.
3. Move your body daily.
4. Savor your meals.
5. Be a qualitarian in the kitchen.
6. Enjoy plant-centric meals.
7. Enjoy healthy fats.
8. Eat fish, mindfully.
9. Embrace plant-based proteins.
10. Eat meat and sweets on occasion.

1. Focus on Food Traditions

Developing a strong food culture through traditions, beliefs, and experiences allows us to have a positive relationship with food, and ultimately to maintain good health.

Tradition Is Good for Your Health

Adopting a Mediterranean diet goes beyond choosing certain foods. It involves the entire eating experience and story behind the food. These rituals and traditions set this diet apart from all others. Supporting evidence: In 2013, UNESCO recognized the Mediterranean diet as an "Intangible Cultural Heritage of Humanity" in an effort to preserve the rituals and traditions of this way of life. In a nutshell, the Mediterranean diet, from its cooking techniques to its farming and agricultural practices, is unique.

How do food traditions impact well-being? By allowing us to:

- Honor our heritage.
- Value our food and the experiences that surround it.
- Protect ourselves against diet culture.
- Recognize the world of flavors that exist in the kitchen.
- Cultivate respect for traditional techniques and culinary craftsmanship.
- Strengthen family ties.
- Celebrate around symbolic meals.

Eat your way through this principle with my favorite seasonal recipes:

Caponata (page 210)

Braised Flat Beans with Tomatoes and Basil (page 132)

Baklava-Style Apple Strudel (page 232)

TIPS FOR FOSTERING POSITIVE FOOD CULTURE AT HOME

- Create your own family traditions—it's never too late to start (make preserves, tomato sauce, or a strawberry pie as a family).
- Spend time with relatives to learn your traditional recipes and cooking methods.
- Discuss food positively at home, not as a tool for weight loss.
- Prepare traditional recipes to highlight festivities.
- Try new foods and restaurants regularly.
- Learn the story behind your recipes and where your ingredients come from.
- Visit markets and shops to discover local products and learn from purveyors.
- Take cooking classes or workshops to learn about a cuisine.

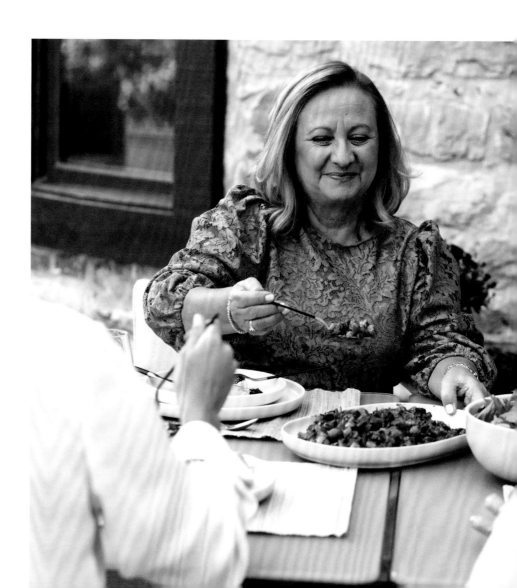

20

2. Share Meals with Loved Ones

The family meal is a daily ritual at the core of the Mediterranean diet. In fact, it's the very base of the Mediterranean Diet Pyramid (page 18), reflecting that how we eat—or, more specifically, who we eat with—is as impactful as what we eat.

The family meal is essential to our well-being because it is:

- A way to communicate and interact with loved ones
- A way to strengthen the family unit and forge new bonds
- A way to preserve cherished culinary traditions
- Associated with better body image in children and adolescents
- Associated with higher academic achievement
- Associated with higher consumption of fruits and vegetables in children

---

TIPS FOR SHARING MEALS

- Get into the habit of eating meals as a family, every day.
- If you live alone, have lunch with a colleague or share a virtual meal with a friend when possible.
- Leave a meal on a friend's doorstep. Nothing puts a smile on someone's face like a homemade meal or baked good.
- Invite the whole family to participate in the menu-planning process.
- Cook as a family.
- Don't wait for holidays to share meals with friends. Long live casual dining!

 Eat your way through this principle with my favorite recipes for gatherings:

Escarole and White Bean Toasts (page 120)

Muhammara (page 108) **with Greek Yogurt Flatbreads** (page 109)

Butternut Squash Lasagna (page 214)

3. Move Your Body Daily

The benefits of physical activity include a lower risk of premature death and chronic disease. Exercise also promotes mental health by improving mood, energy levels, and self-esteem and keeping depressive symptoms at bay, such as feelings of sadness, tiredness, and difficulty sleeping.

How Much Activity Do We Need?

Those living in Mediterranean communities in the 1950s led a way of life that was naturally more active than ours is today. Their daily routines involved hours of walking, gardening, housework, and harvesting, all making for a very active lifestyle. Nowadays, our tasks are more

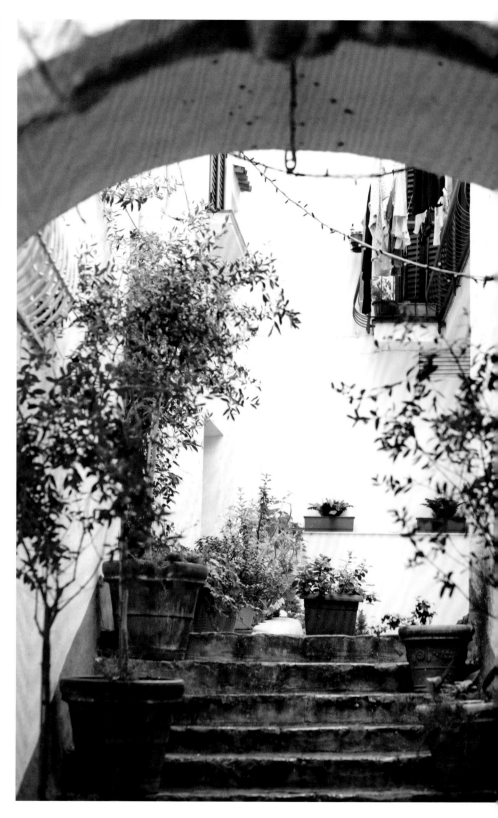

LA PASSEGGIATA: AN ITALIAN RITUAL WORTH ADOPTING

In the evening, many Italians enjoy a stroll with the family through the neighborhood. It's their time to get some fresh air, catch up with friends, and chat.

automated, our work more sedentary. So it takes a conscientious effort to incorporate physical activity into our lifestyle. To be active, according to Canadian guidelines, adults should minimize seated time and also aim to:

- Move at least 2.5 hours (150 minutes) every week.

- Incorporate moderate to vigorous forms of exercise into the week, broken down into 10-minute sessions or longer.

- Include resistance training that targets large muscle groups at least twice per week.

TIPS TO GET MOVING

- Take a family walk after your meal.
- Take your office phone meetings to the street, walking outside when possible.
- Use a sit-stand desk.
- Join a sports team.
- Participate in group activities such as running or walking clubs, or in recreational sports teams.
- Take the stairs instead of the elevator.
- Travel on foot or by bicycle.
- Engage in physical activity that you enjoy. You may have to try several types before you find the right fit.
- Organize your social gatherings around a sport or physical activity (e.g., skiing, hiking, dancing).

---

4. Savor Your Meals

Can you describe the flavors of your most recent meal? In fact, what *do* you recall about the last meal you ate? If you're drawing a blank, you aren't alone. It's become increasingly difficult to incorporate mindful moments in our overstimulated lives, let alone during our meals, meaning that we aren't fully present to enjoy them. But savoring is important for overall meal satisfaction and a key element for a healthy relationship with food. Savor your mealtime by pausing and eating without distraction, and by bringing gratitude to the table for the meal you're about to enjoy. Savor your food by taking small bites, bringing your attention to the aromas, flavors, and textures, as well as to your enjoyment of it.

Slow Down

Mediterranean people are notorious for living la dolce vita. They take their time at the table; rushing a meal is out of the question. Slowing down the

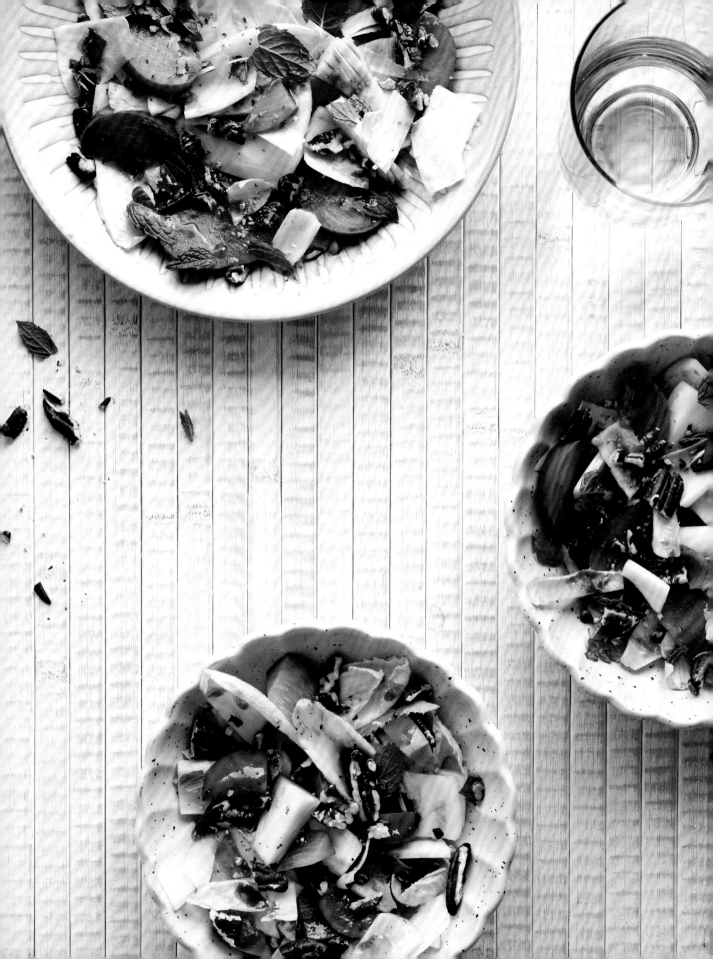

pace allows us to better listen to signals of hunger and satiety. The Mediterranean Diet Pyramid makes no mention of specific portions. That's because, although proportions are important (such as more plant than animal products), the main focus of the pattern is food quality and enjoyment. How much food to eat is left up to the individual to decide. By slowing down, savoring each bite, and deepening our connection to food, we are better able to assess our hunger and satiety cues and fill our plates with what we need. In fact, research shows that taking small bites exposes us to more flavor, which is thought to yield more satisfaction and quicker satiation (a feeling of fullness); this, in turn, results in eating smaller meals.

Tune In

Living in a world without forbidden foods makes it easier to tune in to our body's true wants and reap the most satisfaction from our meals. The Mediterranean diet does not prohibit any foods. Sure, some foods are eaten less often, but every food is allowed. Liberalizing foods in this way helps reduce those relapses caused by food guilt and all-or-nothing tendencies.

TIPS FOR SAVORING YOUR MEALS

- Make the table a no-phone zone. Eat meals without screens on, to minimize distractions.
- Sit down to eat at the table, with a proper place setting, rather than at your desk or on the go.
- Take a deep breath before your meal, and practice gratitude for the meal before you.
- Eat slowly, dedicating 15 to 20 minutes to the meal.
- Chew each bite completely, to fully appreciate the flavors.
- Pay attention to your level of appreciation during a meal.
- Describe each bite, bringing attention to the aroma, flavor, and texture. This keeps you anchored in the eating experience and present to enjoy it.
- Eat when you feel physically hungry. Waiting too long to eat can make it difficult to mindfully savor a meal.
- Stop eating when you reach comfortable fullness (around 80% full).

---

5. Be a Qualitarian in the Kitchen

A tomato, a drizzle of olive oil, and a few torn basil leaves. This trio can taste like heaven as much as it can taste like, well, nothing. Mediterranean cuisine may not be complicated, but it certainly prides itself on using the best ingredients available, to make meals memorable. How can we accomplish this in our day-to-day? By seeking out ingredients that are equal parts nutritious and delicious.

A Nutritious Diet

The Mediterranean diet consists mainly of whole food ingredients or ingredients that are minimally processed and close to their natural state. As foods move up the processing chain, they lose their nutritional integrity. For instance, a bowl of steel-cut oatmeal with fresh blueberries will be more nutritious (and delicious) than a store-bought oat bar with blueberry-flavored filling, and will provide more fiber, micronutrients, and flavor. You may have heard the advice to stay on the perimeter of the store when filling the grocery cart. I don't believe it's always necessary to do that. In fact, there are plenty of processed foods in the center aisles that are highly nutritious and simply made more practical through processing. These products may actually make it easier to stick to a modern Mediterranean diet. Coming back to the oatmeal example, quick-cooking oats and frozen blueberries would be good substitutes for the steel-cut oatmeal and fresh berries, being just as nutritious and perhaps more practical when you're out of time or out of season. Beyond quick-cooking oats and frozen fruit, other examples of nutritious processed foods are dried beans and lentils, frozen vegetables, canned fish, and whole grain breads.

Ultra-processed foods, on the other hand, having moved far up the processing chain, are not only stripped of many of their nutritious elements but have highly palatable ingredients added (the tasty kind that keep you coming back for more, like added sugar, salt, and fat). Ultra-processed are therefore highly manipulated foods and a massive departure from the Mediterranean concept of what food is. In addition, ultra-processed foods are lower in fiber and micronutrients.

A Delicious Diet

Being a qualitarian in the kitchen isn't just about nutrition. Ultimately, it's about being mindful of how your food tastes. From tasting the grapes you buy to adjusting the seasoning while you're cooking, searching for delicious keeps you planted in your eating experience and results in connection with your food and satisfaction from your meal. Fresh fruit and vegetables tend to taste better when they are in season. Of course, in Canada, it's difficult to enjoy our own garden-fresh tomatoes year-round. The Mediterranean diet is about adapting your meal choices so that the end result is as delicious as possible. For instance, I will reserve raw tomato dishes (like Panzanella

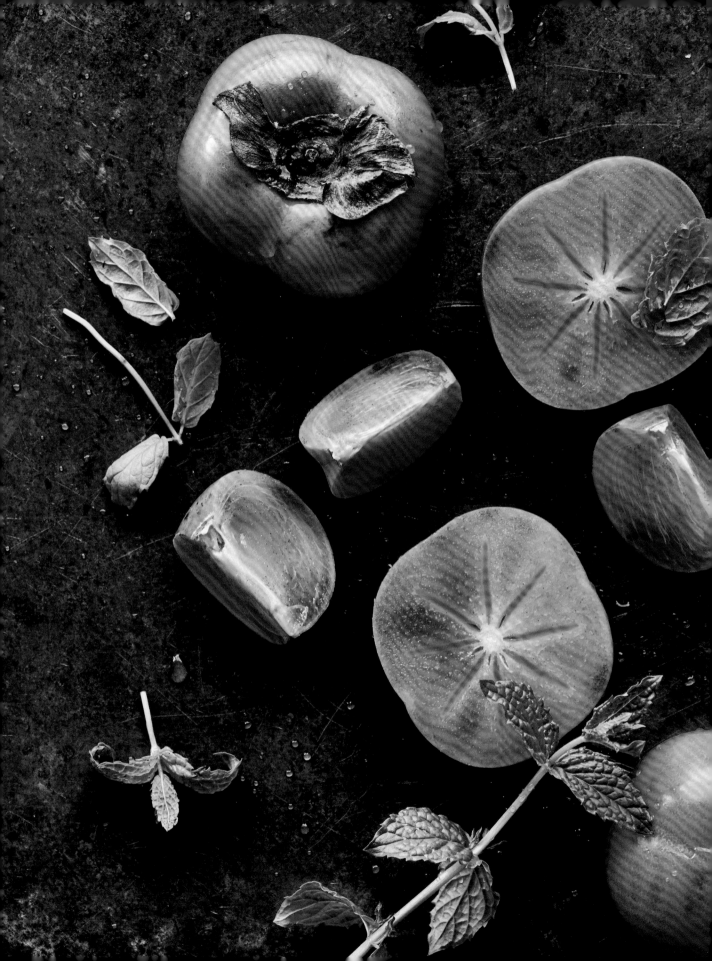

with Avocado, page 90, which uses heirloom tomatoes) for August, opting for a tomato sauce–based dish in the winter. Nutrition should not be the sole motivating factor in the food you choose; flavor quality is just as important to consider. So, if you want ice cream, then allow yourself to fully taste and enjoy the ice cream! Keeping flavor top-of-mind, this experience may look like going to an artisanal shop that uses traditional ice-cream-making techniques or offers creative flavors. Ultimately, an investment in flavor quality and a focus on being intentional with your food choices will yield more enjoyable eating experiences and more satisfaction.

 Eat your way through this principle with these homemade-version recipes:

Classic Pesto (page 248)

Everyday Dressing (page 246)

Marinara Sauce (page 248)

TIPS FOR BEING A QUALITARIAN

- Shop with the seasons, when you can, for more flavorful ingredients.
- Out of season, don't hesitate to use dried or frozen options; frozen is often flash-frozen at peak freshness.
- Take the time to mindfully store your fresh ingredients upon returning from the grocery store, to keep them fresh longer.
- Taste as you cook, observing what you like and dislike.
- Seek out the most flavorful versions of the foods you crave, and make an experience out of it.
- Focus on fresh or minimally processed foods.
- Minimize your intake of ultra-processed foods, which are low in nutritional and flavor value: processed meats, potato chips, breakfast cereals, ice cream, mac and cheese, frozen pizza, soft drinks, commercial juices, and granola bars.
- Explore homemade versions of dressings, marinades, sauces, breadcrumbs, and other basic ingredients, when possible.

---

6. Enjoy Plant-Centric Meals

The Mediterranean diet is not vegetarian per se, but it's composed mostly of plants, usually whole: vegetables, fruits, whole grains, beans, pulses, herbs, and spices. Animal-based foods are generally served on the side.

Powering Up on Plants

These days, nutrition is a hot topic, one in which there's so much conflicting advice that even us professionals get whiplash. But despite conflicting opinions, we can all agree on one thing: for a healthful diet, aim to obtain most of your calories from plants. As we'll discuss in the coming pages, plants are the key to getting enough fiber (a key nutrient found only in plants), micronutrients, and disease-protecting phytonutrients (see Fight-o-Nutrients, page 30). Emerging research suggests that eating a variety of plant foods promotes a diverse microbiome, associated with better health. The microbiome refers to trillions of microorganisms that live in our gut and the way they interact and function in our bodies. Our understanding of this dynamic environment is still limited, but one thing is clear: the microbiome plays an important role in promoting our health. Here are a few ways to get started:

- Fill half of your plate (literally or figuratively) with two fistfuls of vegetables of three colors or more, at least twice per day. For example, enjoy spinach in a morning smoothie, grilled peppers and grilled eggplant in a salad for lunch, and a roasted tomato and leek soup as an appetizer for dinner.

- Add pulses and whole grains to your daily menu. You might have beans with your eggs for breakfast, include farro in your soup for lunch, and accompany a stir-fry with quinoa in the evening.

- Season each meal and snack liberally with herbs and spices. A few ideas: sprinkle cinnamon on your breakfast cereal, add fresh oregano and mint to a salad at lunch, and use cumin, paprika, and crushed chili flakes in a marinade used for dinner.

- Enjoy fresh fruit for dessert—think roasted pears in the winter, apricot cobbler in the spring, grilled peaches in the summer, or a fresh apple in the fall.

Three Reasons to Spice It Up

- Flavor: Herbs and spices (oregano, rosemary, thyme, sage, basil, marjoram, dill, cinnamon, cumin, and coriander, to name a few) are a key element of Mediterranean cuisine, imparting unique and distinguishable flavors.
- Phytochemicals: Herbs and spices are equally if not more nutrient-dense as are fruits and vegetables. Specifically, they're high in phytochemicals that have antioxidant and anti-inflammatory properties.
- Less salt: Herbs and spices are a simple way to add flavor to meals without reaching for the salt shaker.

Fight-o-Nutrients

Phytochemicals are compounds found in high concentrations in brightly colored plants. Although they are not essential nutrients, like vitamins and minerals are, they are beneficial to our health, often because of their antioxidant and anti-inflammatory properties.

Beneficial Plant Compounds and Their Sources in the Mediterranean Diet

FOOD SOURCES	PHYTOCHEMICALS	BIOLOGICAL ACTIVITIES UNDER INVESTIGATION
Broccoli, cabbage, cauliflower, garden cress, kale, watercress	Isothiocyanates	Antibacterial, anticancer, anti-inflammatory, and antioxidant activities
Garlic, leeks, onions, ramps, shallots	Organosulfur compounds	Cardioprotective activities
Apples (all types), berries, broccoli, celery, citrus fruits, chocolate, hot peppers, kale, onions, parsley, red grapes, red wine, scallions, tea (white, green, black, oolong), thyme	Flavonoids	Anti-inflammatory, anti-diabetic, and neuroprotective activities
Berries, eggplant, grapes, red wine	Resveratrol	Cardioprotective activities
Cantaloupe, carrots, dandelion, kale, spinach, peas, pumpkin, squash, tomato paste, tomato purée, watermelon	Carotenoids	Antioxidant potential
Chickpeas, lentils, nuts, olive oil, seeds, whole grains	Phytosterols	Assist in management of cholesterol levels
Asparagus, chicory, fruit (fresh and dried), garlic, pulses, Jerusalem artichokes, onions, cold/reheated rice	Prebiotics	Promote the growth of beneficial gut bacteria and short-chain fatty acid production

Crushing on Color

To encourage people to include a variety of plants in their diet, we dietitians advise to "eat the rainbow." As the chart below shows, each colorful food brings its own benefit. One of the benefits of a colorful Mediterranean diet is the high intake of antioxidants. Think of antioxidants like rust-proofing agents, protecting us against free radicals—unstable molecules that compromise the health of our cells and contribute to aging. Many of these molecules also feed on healthy microbes in our gut. This not only means that eating the rainbow promotes gut health but also that the more colors you incorporate in each plate, the broader the spectrum of healthy bacteria you feed. Aim for three colors per plate at every meal.

EATING THE RAINBOW

RED	Bell peppers, radishes, tomatoes
ORANGE	Bell peppers, carrots, sweet potatoes, winter squash
YELLOW	Beets, corn, tomatoes, zucchini
GREEN	Arugula, asparagus, broccoli, kale, lettuce, spinach, zucchini
PURPLE	Beets, cabbage, eggplant, radicchio
WHITE	Cauliflower, endive, fennel, leeks, mushrooms, onions

Fill Up on Fiber

The Mediterranean diet provides two times more fiber than the standard Western diet, clocking in at 30 grams versus 14 grams per day. Fiber promotes intestinal regularity, helps control blood sugar, and nourishes intestinal microbiota, while reducing the risk of chronic diseases.

TIPS FOR BOOSTING YOUR FIBER INTAKE

- Eat fruits and vegetables with their skin on.
- Add nuts or seeds to your salads.
- Start meals with a mixed green salad.
- Opt for whole grains instead of refined grain products.
- Try new flours—buckwheat, chickpea, almond, spelt.
- Include ground flaxseed in your baking.
- Enjoy a vegetable soup with meals.
- Include whole grain pastas in your pantry.
- Use whole grains like bulgur, brown rice, farro, and whole grain polenta regularly.
- Opt for smoothies instead of juice, to get the full fiber benefit.

Eat your way through this principle with my favorite colorful, high-fiber, and plant-centric recipes:

Dukkah-Crusted Whole Cauliflower (page 166)

Oven-Baked Spinach Falafel (page 158)

Kale Fattoush (page 102)

7. Enjoy Healthy Fats

The olive tree's ability to survive thousands of years in arid climates earned it its legendary reputation as a symbol of peace and longevity. In fact, it is thought that it was the climate that conditioned olive trees to produce such a large number of antioxidants. If, from body care to beauty to cooking, olive oil is considered liquid gold, it's for good reason. As we explore in this chapter, healthy fats like those found in extra virgin olive oil, olives, nuts, and seeds are a key component of the Mediterranean diet.

A High-Fat Diet

One factor that sets the Mediterranean diet apart from other eating patterns is its fat content. Fat contributes more than 35% of calories in the traditional Mediterranean diet, rising to 42% in some regions, including Crete. In contrast, the Canadian recommendations are to provide 20% to 35% of your daily calories from fat. Beyond the amount of fat in a diet, what is most important to consider is where it comes from. The fat in the Mediterranean diet is mainly made up of healthy fats (from monounsaturated fatty acids) because of the high consumption of olive oil. Other regularly eaten sources of monounsaturated fats include nuts, seeds, and whole grain products (which contain the germ). Saturated fats represent only a small proportion of the diet (less than 10%) because of the low consumption of meat, dairy products, and processed foods. Trans fats, known for their harmful effect on cardiovascular health, are not present in the Mediterranean diet.

An Oil Like No Other

Olive oil, essential in Mediterranean cuisine, is thought to be responsible for many of the Mediterranean diet's benefits. Olive oil stands out for its high monounsaturated fat content, beneficial to cardiovascular health. But beyond its fat profile, what makes this precious oil unique is its high content of polyphenols—compounds with antioxidant and anti-inflammatory properties.

Cooking with Olive Oil

If you've browsed the oils section of your grocery store, you have likely seen an array of olive oils. Which is best for everyday cooking? That depends on how well it stands up to heat, and for that, the oil must consist of heat-stable fat, and it must have a high smoke point. Free fatty acids are molecules that are sensitive to oxidation; this is known as the oil's acidity.

The lower the acidity of an oil, the better. All this to say that extra virgin olive oil (EVOO) is the best candidate for everyday cooking, for three reasons. First, it is high in heat-stable monounsaturated fats. Second, it has low acidity and a high smoke point. And finally, it gets its edge thanks to its polyphenol content, antioxidant compounds that not only are responsible for its unique flavor and aroma but that offer added protection against degradation, and add to its stability.

In the chart on page 34, you'll find a breakdown of the most common types of olive oil, plus their best uses in the kitchen. Overall, EVOO is the best choice in the kitchen. It also happens to be my personal preference, for both its health benefits and its flavor. That said, EVOO can break the bank, and fast. Because of its higher price, you might choose to keep two oils on hand: a more neutral-tasting olive oil for everyday cooking, and a high-quality extra virgin olive oil to enjoy raw or when cooking with moderate heat (this will also allow you to fully appreciate its aroma, which is lost with high heat).

How Do Mediterraneans Enjoy Olive Oil?

Mediterraneans enjoy olive oil in several ways:

- By the spoonful! The old Cretan ritual of starting the day with a spoonful of extra virgin olive oil is still practiced today.

- As the main cooking fat.

- Paired with garlic and crushed chili flakes to sauté vegetables in.

- In salad dressings and sauces like pesto and salsa verde.

- Dressing raw vegetables such as tomatoes, cucumbers, and salad greens.

- By dipping country bread into it, to fully appreciate its aroma.

- Drizzled over cooked vegetables such as escarole, rapini, or wild greens.

- In soffritto, the aromatic trio of onion, celery, and carrots that is the base of many Mediterranean dishes.

Types of Olive Oil

TYPE	HOW IT'S MADE	ABOUT THIS OIL	HOW TO USE IT
Extra virgin olive oil (EVOO)	Mechanically extracted from the olive fruit without the use of heat or chemicals, preserving the natural aroma and nutritional integrity of the oil	Low acidity Pronounced flavor High polyphenol content Highest grade of olive oil Most expensive	Highly heat stable, suitable for everyday cooking Due to its higher price and to fully appreciate its aroma that may be lost with high heat, this oil may be best enjoyed raw, such as, in dressings or used for drizzling
Virgin olive oil (VOO)	Mechanically extracted from the olive fruit without the use of heat or chemicals, preserving the natural aroma and nutritional integrity of the oil	Higher acidity than EVOO Mild flavor Less expensive	Lower smoke point than EVOO Sautéing, baking, marinades
Olive oil (refined olive oil) (OO)	Blended with EVOO Mechanical extraction, then refining (bleaching, degumming, deodorizing, neutralizing)	Low acidity Neutral flavor, light color High smoke point Neutral tasting Low to no beneficial polyphenols that EVOO is known for "Light" olive oil is a subset of refined olive oil; "light" refers to the color and flavor Less expensive	High-heat cooking, sautéing, baking

Like a Good Wine

Like wine, extra virgin olive oils have different flavors and aromas, some lighter and others more robust. It's the antioxidants that make each variety unique.

WHEN CHOOSING A QUALITY EXTRA VIRGIN OLIVE OIL, CONSIDER . . .

- OLEIC ACID CONTENT: Choose one that has less than 0.8%.

- DARK BOTTLE: This protects the oil from light.

- HARVEST DATE: This helps gauge freshness. Purchase and consume within 24 months of the harvest date, using within 3 months of opening for maximum freshness.

- ORIGIN: The terms "imported" or "bottled" don't necessarily equate to where the olive oil was sourced. The origin should be stated on the label.

- PRICE: Quality extra virgin olive oil is relatively expensive to produce. Although price is not a guarantee of quality, beware if it falls below $15 per 3 cups (750 mL), especially if the product is not supported by the other factors mentioned above.

- TASTE: Have fun sampling the oils. Observe how the aroma and flavor change from one region to another. Some are grassy, some fruity, others peppery. Choose the one you like best, or collect a few and have fun pairing them with various ingredients.

- CERTIFICATION (BONUS): Olive oil is among the most fraudulent products. There are numerous certifying bodies that will put their stamp on products that have been verified for quality and authenticity. Consider this a bonus, though: certification is not mandatory, and it can be a costly process for the producer.

Eat your way through this principle with these recipes high in healthy fats:

Creamy Farfalle Pasta Salad with Artichoke Hearts (page 164)

Sweet and Savory Roasted Nuts with Rosemary and Honey (page 111)

Cherry, Cacao, and Olive Oil Smoothie (page 74)

8. Eat Fish, Mindfully

Fishing is part of the Mediterranean culture, with fish and seafood appearing regularly on the menu—usually at least twice per week if not more. Fish and seafood are excellent sources of protein and can contribute important nutrients to the diet, including vitamin B12, vitamin D, iodine, iron, and selenium. In addition, certain types of fish represent the best dietary sources of the omega-3 fatty acids EPA and DHA—beneficial fats that play a fundamental role in brain development, heart health, and more. On the other hand, the health risks of methylmercury exposure from fish consumption may be a concern. To avoid excessive intake, Canadian guidelines suggest limiting consumption of larger fish like those listed on page 36, in which mercury tends to accumulate more significantly. Finally, when it comes to fresh versus frozen, keep in mind that the nutritional

🌿 Eat your way through this principle with these seafood-based recipes:

Mackerel Bucatini with Crispy Anchovy Breadcrumbs (page 176)

Baked Salmon with Gremolata Crust (page 182)

Cod, Spinach, and Chickpea Casserole (page 174)

content is the same. Unless the fresh option at the fish counter truly is fresh, go ahead and opt for frozen varieties, which are flash-frozen at sea upon catching.

Which Seafood to Choose?

- Fish with high levels of omega-3 fats (EPA and DHA) while also being low in mercury include anchovy, Atlantic mackerel, char, herring, rainbow trout, salmon, and sardines.
- Fish and seafood that are high in protein and relatively low in fat include cod, crab, haddock, hake, halibut, scallops, and shrimp.
- Health Canada recommends to limit high-mercury fish—escolar, marlin, orange roughy, shark, swordfish, and tuna—to 150 grams in total per week for the general population or 150 grams in total per month for those who may become pregnant or are breastfeeding.

A Word on Sustainable Fishing

The state of the oceans when the Mediterranean diet came to researchers' attention more than 50 years ago was very different from what it is today. We must make conscious choices about fish if we want to give our children the chance to enjoy the taste of the sea too. Unfortunately, our bringing fish from the ocean to the plate has non-negligible ecological consequences: overfishing, accidental catches, and destruction of natural habitats. Ask your fishmonger questions, especially what local options are available, so that you can make informed choices. Look for logos from organizations like the Marine Stewardship Council (MSC), which is just one organization whose certification guarantees that the product is sustainably sourced. Also, don't overlook frozen or canned options for fish; these are often less expensive than their fresh counterpart and just as tasty. (I keep canned tuna, salmon, mackerel, sardines, and herring.)

9. Embrace Plant-Based Proteins

The protein intake in the traditional Mediterranean diet is about 20% lower than that of the modern Western diet. The majority of this intake comes from plant sources, including pulses and whole grains. Yogurt, cheese, poultry, and eggs are also on the menu but are generally eaten in small quantities. The key message here is to not depend solely on the animal kingdom to meet your protein needs. By varying your food sources and embracing new foods, it is possible to obtain a wide range of nutrients.

Protein Content of Plant Foods

FOOD	SERVING SIZE	PROTEIN (GRAMS)
Chickpea pasta, dry	3 oz (85 g)	17
Chickpeas, cooked	¾ cup (180 mL)	11
Green peas, cooked	¾ cup (180 mL)	7
Kidney beans, cooked	¾ cup (180 mL)	11
Lentils, cooked	¾ cup (180 mL)	18
Lima beans, cooked	¾ cup (180 mL)	11
Lupini beans, cooked	¾ cup (180 mL)	20
Nuts, mixed	¼ cup (60 mL)	7
Red lentil pasta, dry	3 oz (85 g)	20
Vegetables, mixed	½ cup (125 mL)	3

Cooking Guidelines for Pulses

PULSE	QUANTITY, DRY	SOAKING REQUIRED?	COOKING TIME	YIELD
Beans	1 cup (250 mL)	Yes	1½–2 hours	2½ cups (625 mL)
Chickpeas	1 cup (250 mL)	Yes	1½–2 hours	2½ cups (625 mL)
Split peas	1 cup (250 mL)	No	45 minutes	2 cups (500 mL)
Whole lentils	1 cup (250 mL)	No	20–30 minutes	2½ cups (625 mL)
Split lentils	1 cup (250 mL)	No	10–15 minutes	2 cups (500 mL)

Cooking with Dried Pulses

Most of the recipes in the book can be made with canned beans, chickpeas, or lentils, as these are quick, practical, and nutritionally equivalent to their dried counterparts. However, if you have the time, cook dried pulses from scratch—you won't be disappointed. The process is easy and yields better texture and flavor than canned versions. Here's how to do it:

Soaking Method

1. Rinse the pulses in a colander, removing any that are shrivelled, along with any pebbles or other debris.
2. Place the pulses in a large bowl and cover with cold water. Use 3 cups (750 mL) water for every 1 cup (250 mL) dried pulses. Let stand 12 hours or overnight in the refrigerator.
3. Drain the pulses and rinse thoroughly. This will eliminate some of the indigestible sugars that can cause uncomfortable gas.
4. Transfer the pulses to a large pot and cover with 2 inches (5 cm) water. Feel free to add aromatics to impart flavor—I like bay leaf, onion, carrot, and celery. Season with salt, bring to a boil, and then reduce to a simmer. Cook until the pulses have a slightly firm bite but creamy texture, following the guidelines on page 38.
5. Once cooked, drain and use in your favorite recipes.
6. Store cooked pulses in an airtight container in the refrigerator for up to 4 days or in the freezer for up to 6 months.

🍃 Eat your way through this principle with these pulse-powered recipes:

Roasted Tomato and Lentil Soup with Halloumi Croutons (page 88)

Spiced Roasted Chickpeas (page 110)

Farro e Fagioli (page 86)

10. Eat Meat and Sweets on Occasion

Red Meat on the Side

In the Mediterranean, red meat was traditionally not as accessible as poultry or fish was, and it was also more expensive. As a result, red meat was eaten only occasionally—a few times a month. Today we have better access to red meat, but we also face environmental issues that lead us to the conclusion that eating more plants is better for both our health and for the planet. Using red meat as a side dish rather than the main course or as a food to mark special occasions is a simple way to moderate your consumption.

No Forbidden Foods

Desserts and sweets are on the menu every week in the Mediterranean diet, especially on special occasions and for large family gatherings. On a daily basis, though, fruit is served after meals.

🍃 Eat your way through this principle with the help of a few of my favorite recipes:

Flourless Chocolate, Hazelnut, and Espresso Cake (page 226)

Flank Steak Salad with Crispy White Beans (page 204)

Chocolate Chip and Almond Cantuccini (page 228)

Where Does Your Glass of Vino Fit In?

In the traditional Mediterranean diet, red wine is consumed regularly but in moderation. That is to say, red wine regularly accompanies the meal, but the glass size is kept small (think small juice glass, not oversized wine glass), with one to two drinks, at most, consumed per occasion. Although red wine is an integral part of the traditional diet, consuming alcohol is not without risk. According to a 2018 report by the World Cancer Research Fund, there is strong evidence to suggest that alcohol consumption at any level increases the risk of cancers. And so, if you aren't in the habit of enjoying a glass of red wine with meals, there's no need to start. In fact, the 2023 report of Canada's Guidance on Alcohol and Health echoed this by setting the recommendation for two standard drinks per week, to likely avoid any alcohol-related consequences.

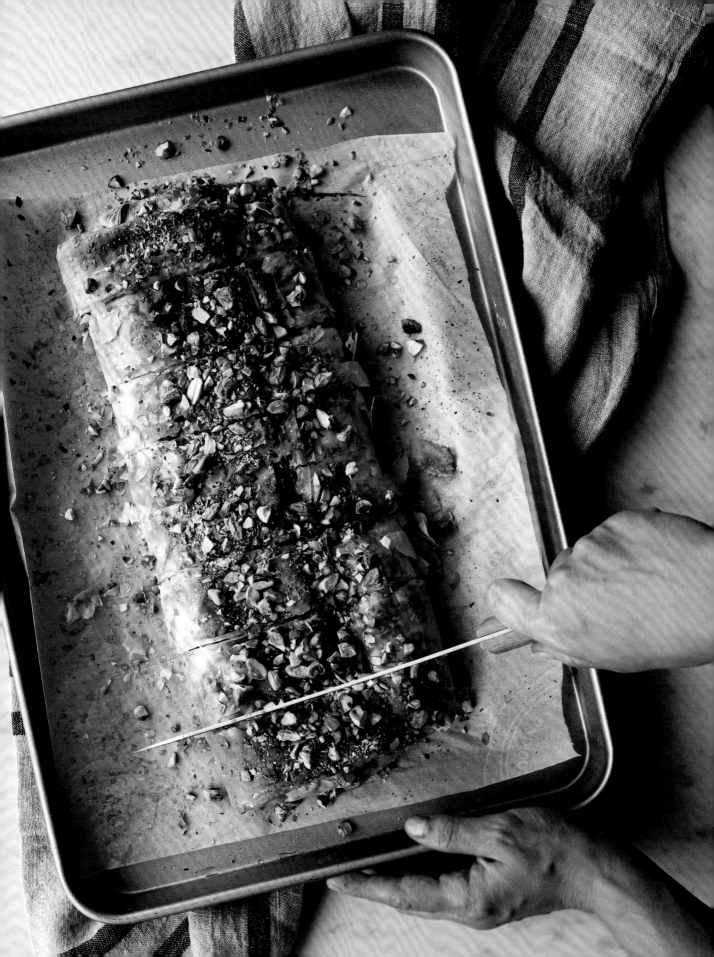

The Benefits

For decades, the body of evidence linking the Mediterranean diet to positive health outcomes has been growing. The benefits of this eating pattern were first documented in the pioneering Seven Countries Study (SCS), led by American scientist Ancel Keys. He and his team linked the diet of those living in Crete and Southern Italy to better health. This discovery led to coining of the term "Mediterranean diet," a diet scientists have been looking at ever since.

An Overview

How does the Mediterranean diet work its magic? The exact mechanism is unknown, mainly because it's impossible to isolate a single food or nutrient as the source of its benefits. It's the harmonic combination of its components that is likely the cause. In this chapter, I outline the primary health outcomes of a traditional Mediterranean diet.

BENEFITS ASSOCIATED WITH THE MEDITERRANEAN DIET

- Reduced overall mortality
- Reduced risk of cardiovascular diseases
- Reduced risk of cancer
- Protection against type 2 diabetes and its complications
- Reduced risk of dementia, including Alzheimer's disease

- Reduced risk of depression
- Improved fertility
- Improved quality of life for people with osteoarthritis
- Protection against asthma
- And more

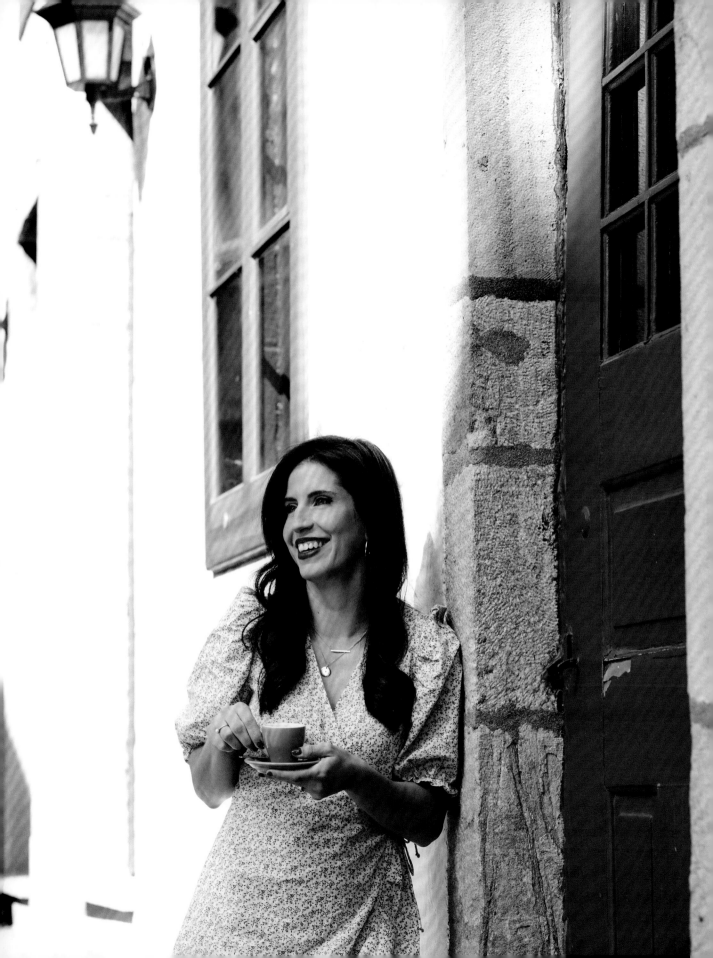

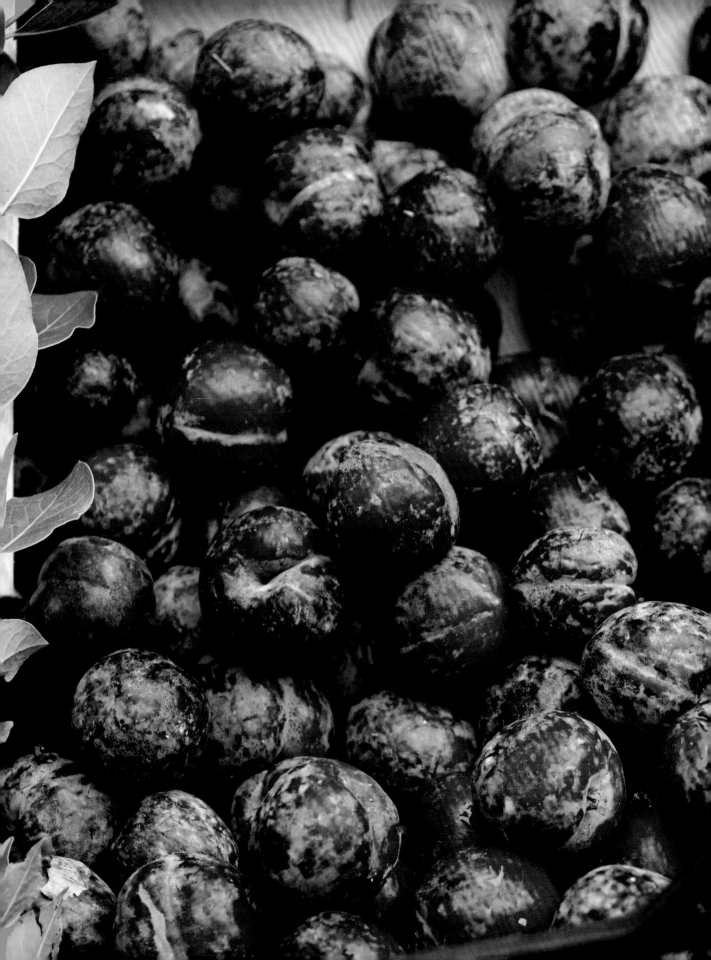

Longevity

One of the most consistent benefits associated with the Mediterranean eating pattern is increased life expectancy. In an extensive review pooling data from multiple studies and over 12 million subjects, the link between the Mediterranean diet and lower mortality risk was so convincing that it was deemed "robust."

Not-So-Secret Ingredient

It's tempting to want to isolate and bottle up a single ingredient from the Mediterranean fountain of youth. Unfortunately, as I've mentioned, no one food is responsible for the diet's rejuvenating effect. In fact, beyond the food, the social dimension of the Mediterranean diet, which sets it apart from other popular diets, appears to be a critical factor in followers' longevity. Researchers agree that living a life surrounded by loved ones is essential for aging in good health and slowing cognitive decline.

Turning Back the Clock

Biological aging occurs for many reasons: aging cells, oxidative damage, and telomere shortening. Telomeres are like hubcaps on the ends of our chromosomes, which shorten during our lifetime. It's believed that telomere shortening may cause aging and age-related diseases, and that our diets play a part in slowing down that process. High adherence to the Mediterranean diet is associated with longer telomeres and thus delayed biological aging.

Defining Aging

Aging is a natural part of life and the result of our body's response to the stressors it faces over our lifetime. Our body aging can be described in various ways:

- Unsuccessful aging: The development of age-related diseases and decline in physical and cognitive function.
- Successful aging: Defined by the World Health Organization as developing and maintaining the functional ability that enables well-being in older age. In a nutshell, it means aging and staying independent, despite having some health conditions.
- Healthy aging: Refers to aging while preserving physical and cognitive health without disease.

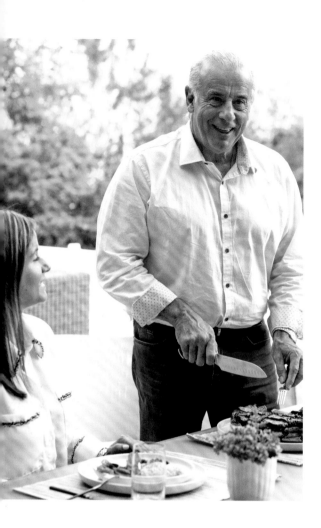

Adding Life to Our Years

The HALE (Healthy Aging: A Longitudinal Study in Europe) project followed healthy elderly men and women aged 70 and older. The results showed that sticking with a Mediterranean diet resulted in a 50% lower mortality risk. What's more, this dietary pattern is also strongly associated with *healthy* aging, described as living to 70 years or older with no significant chronic disease and in good physical and mental health. Aging is unavoidable, so why not age in good health?

It's no surprise that diet quality is considered the leading modifiable cause of death and disability worldwide. That's because food and lifestyle habits are key determinants in the aging process. The Mediterranean diet includes these healthy habits:

- Physical activity
- High consumption of plant-based proteins
- Low intake of trans fats and saturated fat
- Low intake of refined carbohydrates
- High intake of fruit and vegetables
- High intake of foods rich in vitamins, minerals, micronutrients, and bioactive compounds

Heart Health

Ever since the first observational data from the Seven Countries Study, linking the Mediterranean lifestyle to the lowest rates of heart disease at the time, cardiovascular health remains the most widely researched benefit of the diet. Today, the evidence is vast and consistent: the Mediterranean diet is associated with better cardiovascular health outcomes than are other dietary patterns. The Lyon Diet Heart Study was a landmark trial—it was the first randomized trial to show a strong cardiovascular protection from a dietary intervention. This study assigned participants with known coronary artery disease to a Mediterranean diet or a low-fat control diet. The study found that participants following the Mediterranean diet saw a 50% to 70% lower risk of recurrent heart disease two years after follow-up, compared to those following the low-fat diet. From the PREDIMED trial, a study whose participants were at high risk for heart disease, researchers concluded that

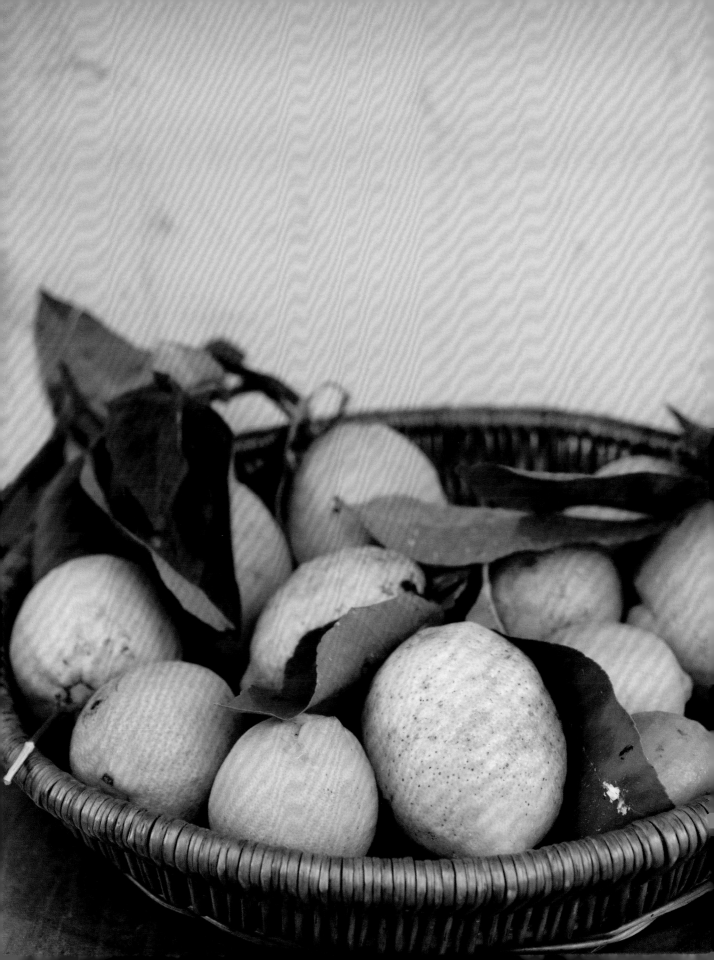

a Mediterranean diet supplemented with olive oil or nuts significantly reduced the incidence of major cardiovascular events compared with a low-fat diet.

Diabetes

It is estimated that, by the year 2050, one in three people will be affected by type 2 diabetes, despite it being preventable through lifestyle change. The Mediterranean diet improves glycemic control and insulin sensitivity and is recommended to prevent adult-onset type 2 diabetes. In a prospective cohort study of over 13,000 participants, sticking with a Mediterranean diet reduced the risk of developing type 2 diabetes by 83%.

Cancer

In a recent study, adherence to a Mediterranean diet was associated with reduced death from overall cancer and the risk of developing certain cancers. It is suspected that the high presence of plant-based foods on the Mediterranean menu is responsible for its protective effect, since these foods provide high amounts of fiber and antioxidants. As well, the Mediterranean diet also promotes regular physical activity, a low consumption of red and processed meats, and a moderate alcohol consumption, habits that are known to reduce cancer risk.

Mental Health

When researchers studied the Mediterranean diet and clinical depression, they found that it significantly lowered the risk of developing depressive symptoms. This is thought to be because of the anti-inflammatory nature of the diet and the plant-heavy cuisine. Beyond the plate, the community component is at the heart of the Mediterranean diet, emphasizing family meals and conviviality. These factors are also recognized as supportive for mental health, by preserving cognitive functions like memory, language, and understanding, and by warding off loneliness.

Fertility

While there is no single "fertility diet," the Mediterranean diet is a balanced and beneficial option for couples wishing to conceive. Rich in plants and low in processed foods, the Mediterranean diet provides many fertility-supporting nutrients, notably its high monounsaturated fat content, which plays a crucial role in ovulatory health, and its high anti-oxidant content, which may help protect reproductive cells from damage. Couples wanting to conceive might consider adopting the diet at least 3 to 6 months in advance.

Fertility and the Mediterranean Diet

Assisted reproductive treatment	Adopting a Mediterranean diet before IVF treatment may increase the chance of pregnancy.
Male fertility	A Mediterranean diet was linked to better sperm-quality parameters, particularly concentration and motility.
Polycystic ovary syndrome (PCOS)	PCOS is the most common hormonal disorder affecting women of childbearing age, and it is a cause of infertility because of ovulation issues. Research shows the Mediterranean diet plays a part in managing PCOS-related symptoms, thanks to its effect on insulin resistance, inflammation, and hyperandrogenism.

Going Mediterranean Every Day

The beauty of the Mediterranean eating pattern is that you don't have to travel farther than the grocery store to adopt its principles. But how do we fit the diet into our hectic lives? The key is to modernize the traditional Mediterranean by equipping yourself with a few strategies.

Change, Slowly but Surely

As a dietitian, I work with individuals eager to completely transform their lives. They are often surprised when I ask them to slow down—because when it comes to building healthy habits that last, we often need to slow down to get ahead. Your health will see a more significant change if you adopt one new habit every week for the next year than if you were to overhaul your diet overnight, only to burn out in a month. Here's a list of buildable habits to get you started:

- Use olive oil as your main cooking fat (see page 34 for how to choose an olive oil).
- Replace one meat-based meal per week with a plant-based one.
- Add nuts, seeds, or olives to salads, or enjoy as a snack a few times per week.
- Enjoy a green salad with an olive oil–based dressing as a side to your lunch or dinner.
- Try new whole grains, such as brown rice or farro, or whole grain flours when baking.
- Cook one (or more!) Mediterranean recipe from this book every week.

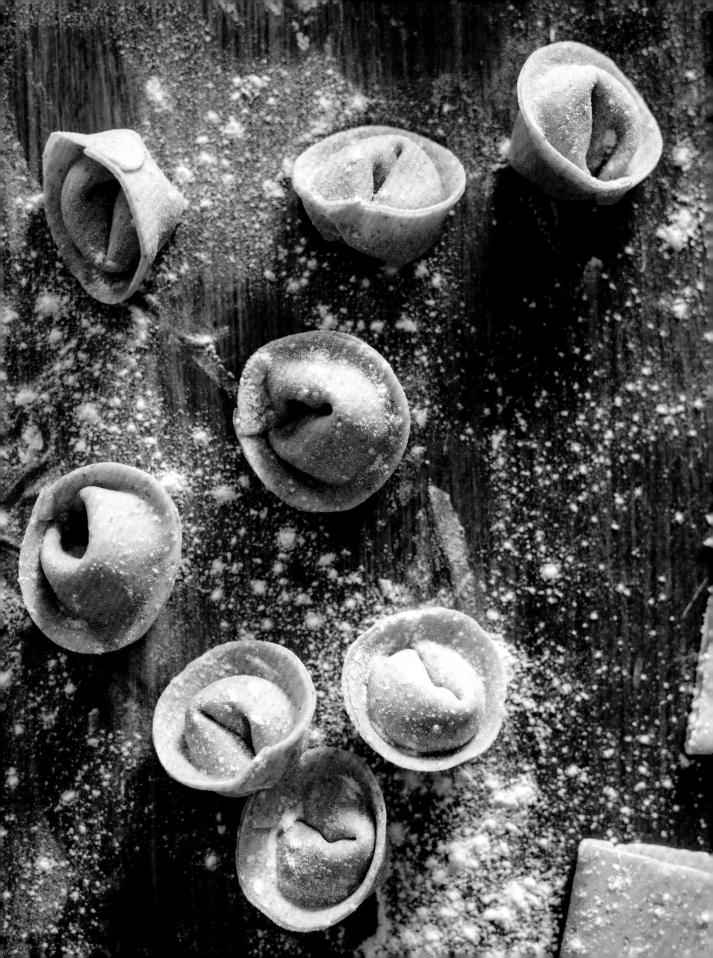

- Visit a Mediterranean specialty store and purchase herbs, spices, or condiments to try.
- Add beans, chickpeas, and lentils to your favorite dishes, including soups, salads, and snacks.

Meal Prep

There's no right or wrong way to meal prep in the Mediterranean diet. Whether you choose to batch-cook simple ingredients to mix and match later in the week, or prefer stocking your refrigerator with complete meals, you always come out a winner when you cook in advance. Set aside 30 to 60 minutes per week for this practice to lighten the Monday-through-Friday meal routine. Below are examples of simple ingredients and dishes to prepare in advance.

Simple Meal-Prep Ideas

VEGETABLES

Grilled, blanched, or steamed vegetables

Salad mix (washed, drained)

Vegetable platter

Vegetable soup

Peeled garlic for the week

WHOLE GRAINS OR PULSES

Brown rice

Oven-Baked Spinach Falafel (page 158)

Greek Yogurt Flatbreads (page 109)

Farro (to be used in Warm Mushroom, Farro, and Radicchio Salad, page 92, or in Mediterranean Farro and Chickpea Bowl, page 148)

Sumac Bean Salad (page 155)

EGGS OR MEATS

Hard-boiled eggs (to be used in Tuna, Egg, and Potato Salad, page 94)

Chicken patties (to be used in the Greek Chicken Burgers, page 206)

Zucchini and Ricotta Sformato (page 160)

CONDIMENTS

Marinara sauce (page 248)

Salad dressing (page 246)

Classic Pesto (page 248)

Salsa Verde (page 250)

Tahini Sauce (page 249)

Menu Planning

Although I'm a big believer in the weekly meal-prep session, sometimes it just isn't in the cards, and that's okay! In those instances, menu planning is well worth your time. Having a game plan guides you as the week progresses, ultimately helping you avoid the dreaded "What's for dinner?" question.

Begin by looking at your calendar for the week ahead and selecting recipes based on upcoming activities, family preferences, and grocery specials you want to take advantage of. Plug the recipes into your menu plan, using dinner leftovers for lunch the next day whenever possible, for even more efficiency. See page 54 for a complete weekly meal plan.

A Well-Stocked Kitchen

To cook good food, you must have good food on hand. Keeping the kitchen stocked with the essentials will make a world of difference when it comes to preparing quick, nourishing meals. This section showcases the categories I consider essential for a well-stocked kitchen, along with lists of some of my favorite ingredients—which aren't must-haves, but rather nice-to-haves. In other words, feel free to explore these suggestions and build them into your kitchen gradually. Keeping a variety of these foods on hand truly simplifies the task of creating flavorful and nourishing meals.

Vegetables and Fruits

Since vegetables and fruits play a big part in the Mediterranean meal, they should fill the majority of your grocery cart. Focus, as much as possible, on what is local and seasonal. And remember that frozen fruits and vegetables are just as nutritious as fresh. So the next time you shop, consider putting these items in your cart:

- **Fresh herbs:** basil, dill, mint, oregano, parsley, rosemary, thyme
- **Fresh produce (choosing options from each color group makes it easy to eat the rainbow at every meal):**
  - **Green:** arugula, asparagus, broccoli, Brussels sprouts, celery, cucumber, kale, lime, rapini, romaine, spinach, string beans, Swiss chard
  - **Red and purple:** beets, berries, cabbage, eggplant, grapes, peppers, plums, radicchio, radishes, tomatoes, watermelon
  - **Yellow and orange:** butternut squash, cantaloupe, carrots, clementines, lemons, mangoes, oranges, sweet potatoes

Mediterranean Diet Meal Plan

	BREAKFAST	LUNCH	SNACK	DINNER
MONDAY	Bruschetta-Style Pea and Avocado Toast (page 78)	Mediterranean Farro and Chickpea Bowl (page 148)	Seasonal fruit Cucumber Dill and Avocado Hummus (page 106)	Baked Salmon with Gremolata Crust (page 182) Fennel and Orange Salad (page 96)
TUESDAY	Yogurt Raspberries Fig and Olive Oil Granola (page 68)	Roasted Tomato and Lentil Soup with Halloumi Croutons (page 88)	Seasonal fruit Spiced Roasted Chickpeas (page 110)	Moroccan Squash and Chickpea Stew (page 156)
WEDNESDAY	Egg and Halloumi Breakfast Plate (page 80)	Moroccan Squash and Chickpea Stew (page 156)	Seasonal fruit Olives with Fennel and Chili (page 114)	Cod in Fennel Broth (page 178)
THURSDAY	Cherry, Cacao, and Olive Oil Smoothie (page 74)	Roasted Tomato and Lentil Soup with Halloumi Croutons (page 88)	Seasonal fruit Sweet and Savory Roasted Nuts with Rosemary and Honey (page 111)	Greek Chicken Burgers (page 206)
FRIDAY	Yogurt Raspberries Fig and Olive Oil Granola (page 68)	Greek Chicken Burgers (page 206)	Seasonal fruit Lupini beans	Farro e Fagioli (page 86)
SATURDAY	Bruschetta-Style Pea and Avocado Toast (page 78)	Farro e Fagioli (page 86)	Seasonal fruit Figgy Walnut Energy Bites (page 236)	Kale Fattoush (page 102) Oven-Baked Spinach Falafel (page 158)
SUNDAY	Egg, Lima Bean, and Feta Breakfast Skillet (page 76)	Oven-Baked Spinach Falafel (page 158)	Seasonal fruit Celery and anchovies	Antipasto Mackerel Bucatini with Crispy Anchovy Breadcrumbs (page 176) Chocolate Chip and Almond Cantuccini (page 228)

- **White**: bananas, cauliflower, endive, garlic, leeks, mushrooms, onions, potatoes
- **Frozen produce**: blueberries, broccoli, cherries, spinach, strawberries
- **Pantry vegetables (store in a cool dark place)**: onions, garlic, ginger, potatoes, shallots, sweet potatoes, tomatoes, winter squash (acorn, butternut, spaghetti)
- **Tomatoes, canned**: diced, and whole peeled
- Tomato purée (tomato passata)
- Tomato paste (buy it in a tube, for convenience)

Whole Grains and Flour-Based Products

Versatile and highly nutritious, whole grains can be used in salads, soups, pilafs, or even as the basis of a stir-fry. They absorb the flavors of your dishes, making them even more delicious. Here are some I like to keep on hand:

- Bulgur
- **Couscous**: Israeli and whole grain
- Farro
- **Flours**: all-purpose, buckwheat, chickpea, oat, spelt, whole wheat
- **Oats**: quick-cooking (for baking), rolled oats (for granola), and steel-cut (for porridge) (Opt for plain, unsweetened oats and flavor them yourself.)
- **Pasta**: an array of shapes, sizes, and flours, including chickpea, lentil, spelt, and white
- Polenta
- Quinoa
- **Rice**: short-grain varieties (risotto, brown), black, and long-grain

---

Whole Grain Tips

- Store dried whole grains in a cool, dry place for up to 6 months.
- Rinse the grains thoroughly before cooking.
- Store cooked grains like rice, farro, quinoa, and bulgur in the freezer for up to 6 months (for meal prep!).

Pulses

Beans, chickpeas, lentils, and peas are nutritional powerhouses, versatile and affordable, so it's no wonder they are the core of so many Mediterranean recipes. Buy them canned or dried, depending on how much time you can afford to prepare them.

- **Beans (canned and/or dried):** black, cranberry, lima, lupini (the jarred ones are great for snacking), white (cannellini)
- **Chickpeas:** canned, dried (for falafel, page 158), and roasted (for snacking)
- **Lentils:** dried French (Puy), dried red
- **Pulse flour and products:**
  - Chickpea flour
  - Pulse-flour pasta: chickpea pasta, red lentil pasta, pea pasta

> **Pulse Tips**
> - Gradually increase your consumption over time if you are not used to eating beans.
> - Store dried pulses in a cool, dry place for up to 12 months.
> - Store cooked beans in the freezer for up to 6 months.

Dried Fruit

You can use dried fruit in both savory and sweet dishes. Choose versions without added sugar and oil.

- Apricots
- Cherries
- **Dates:** Medjool, Deglet Nour
- Figs
- Raisins

Dried Herbs and Spices

These are staples of Mediterranean cuisine, and dried spices are essential for bringing your dishes to life. You'll get the most of a spice's aroma if you buy it whole.

- Bay leaves
- Black peppercorns

- **Chili:** dried whole chilis, crushed chili flakes, ground cayenne pepper
- Cinnamon
- Cloves
- Coriander seeds
- Cumin
- Fennel seeds
- Ginger (ground)
- Mint (dried)
- Nutmeg
- Oregano (dried)
- **Paprikas:** sweet, smoked
- Salt
- Sumac
- Thyme (dried)
- Za'atar

Spice Tips

- Buy whole spices when possible—they will last longer and offer more flavor than other forms.
- Store spices in a dark and cool place.

Oils and Vinegars

- Apple cider vinegar
- Balsamic vinegar
- Extra virgin olive oil
- Red wine vinegar
- Sherry vinegar
- White wine vinegar

For Drinking

- Coffee (ground)
- Espresso beans
- **Teas:** green, black, chamomile, peppermint, fennel, dandelion root

Nuts and Seeds

Nuts and seeds are packed with the healthy trifecta of fat, fiber, and protein, along with other nutrients. They also add texture to a dish. This makes them ideal for snacking and baking in both sweet and savory dishes alike. Try Sweet and Savory Roasted Nuts with Rosemary and Honey (page 111).

- Almonds
- Chia seeds
- Coconut
- Flaxseed
- Hazelnuts
- Hemp seeds
- Pecans
- Pistachios
- Sesame seeds
- Walnuts

Nut and Seed Tips

- Purchase unsalted if you can, otherwise the sodium content can be quite high.
- Store a small portion in your pantry, but if buying in bulk, store the majority in the refrigerator or freezer, in an airtight jar or bag, to keep them fresh. They will keep in the freezer for up to 1 year.

Condiments and Canned Goods

- Artichoke hearts, canned in water
- Chili oil
- Crushed hot peppers in oil
- Eggplant pickled in olive oil
- Harissa
- Honey
- **Fish**: canned sardines, mackerel, and tuna
- Maple syrup (pure)
- **Mustard**: Dijon and whole grain
- **Olives**: jarred or salt-cured
- **Roasted red peppers**: jarred and water-packed
- **Turnips**: pickled in water

Mindful Cooking

To reap the many benefits of the Mediterranean diet, you must practice one habit daily: cooking. Cooking bridges the gap between food and nourishment. It turns your nutrition knowledge into behaviors that make a real impact on your health. It brings people together and helps honor precious traditions. In Part Two: The Recipes (page 65), I share my recipes based on this traditional diet; some are inspired by my family heritage, others involve my favorite flavors. I also provide you with practical tips to use every day. My ultimate goal is to inspire you to cook, so you may eat your way through the principles in this book and make every day Mediterranean.

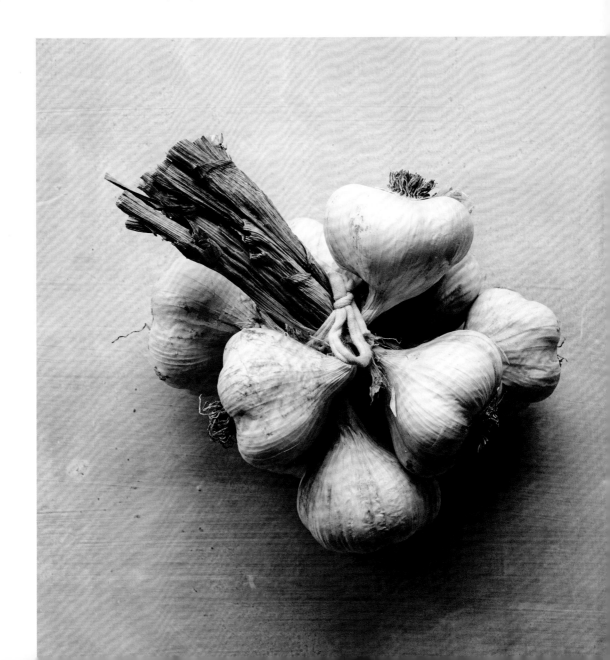

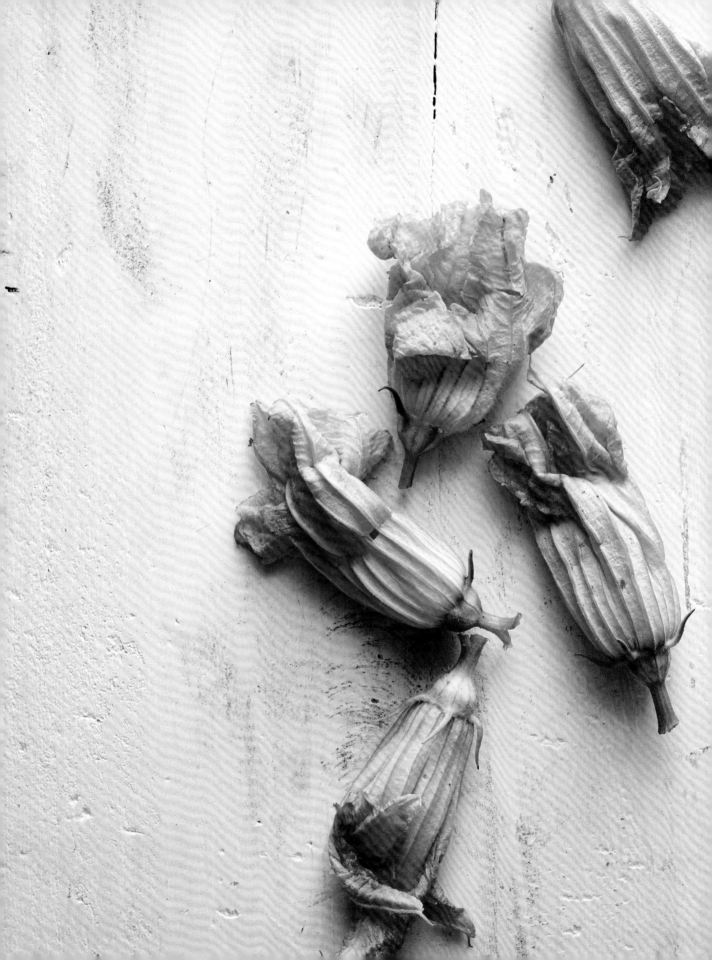

How to Use This Book

A few notes before we get cooking. Some of the recipes in this book recommend using a convection oven setting because the convection setting blows air in a continuous fashion, making for even cooking and achieving crispy, baked-not-fried results. If you do not have this setting, you can increase the listed temperature by 25°F. You will also notice that salt is left "to taste" in the recipes. I've always found salting to be an individual preference and best left to you and your palate. Plus, it's all the more reason to enjoy the process of cooking and taste as you go. Finally, you will notice labels listed for each recipe. Here is what they mean:

Vegan: Recipe with no animal products or honey
Vegetarian: Recipe is meat-free, but may still contain fish, dairy, and/or eggs
Dairy-free*: Recipe contains no dairy products
Gluten-free*: Recipe contains no wheat, barley, or rye
Nut-free*: Recipe contains no peanuts or tree nuts

*For celiac disease or severe allergies, always check ingredient lists of individual products (for instance, oats or spices) to ensure no traces will be present.

Mediterranean Diet at a Glance

Nutritional Characteristics of the Mediterranean Diet

- High intake of monounsaturated fat, from extra virgin olive oil, nuts, seeds, tahini, and avocado.
- High complex carbohydrate intake from grains and pulses.
- High fiber intake from vegetables and fruit.
- High phytochemical intake from plant-based foods (oils, nuts, vegetables, herbs, fruit).

An Overview of the Lifestyle and Dietary Habits of the Mediterranean Diet

Lifestyle and Culture

- Food traditions, preserving traditions, and cooking regularly.
- Meal sharing and conviviality.
- Quality, seasonality, and eco-friendliness.
- **Movement:** Regular physical activity at least 30 minutes daily.

Dietary

Daily

- **Cold-pressed extra virgin olive oil**: To be used as the primary source of dietary fat with meals.
- **Grains and pulses**: Whole grains and pulses like beans, chickpeas, and lentils, often as the base of meals.
- **Vegetables**: Two fistfuls per plate of three colors or more, at least twice per day.
- **Fruit**: Two to three servings daily, fresh and often eaten as a dessert.
- **Herbs and spices**: Use liberally in meals to optimize flavor.
- **Water**: Your drink of choice. Aim for 6 to 8 glasses, or more, depending on your level of physical activity, to ensure proper hydration.

Regularly

- **Nuts, seeds, olives**: Great for snacking, these contribute to healthy fat intake. Enjoy at least three times per week.
- **Fish and shellfish**: Two or more servings weekly, being mindful of fishing practices.
- **Dairy, poultry, and eggs**: Eaten weekly to daily.

Occasionally

- **Red meat and processed meat**: Eaten on a monthly basis, or less.
- **Sweets, cakes, or pastries**: To be enjoyed on a weekly basis.

PART TWO

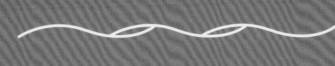

The
Recipes

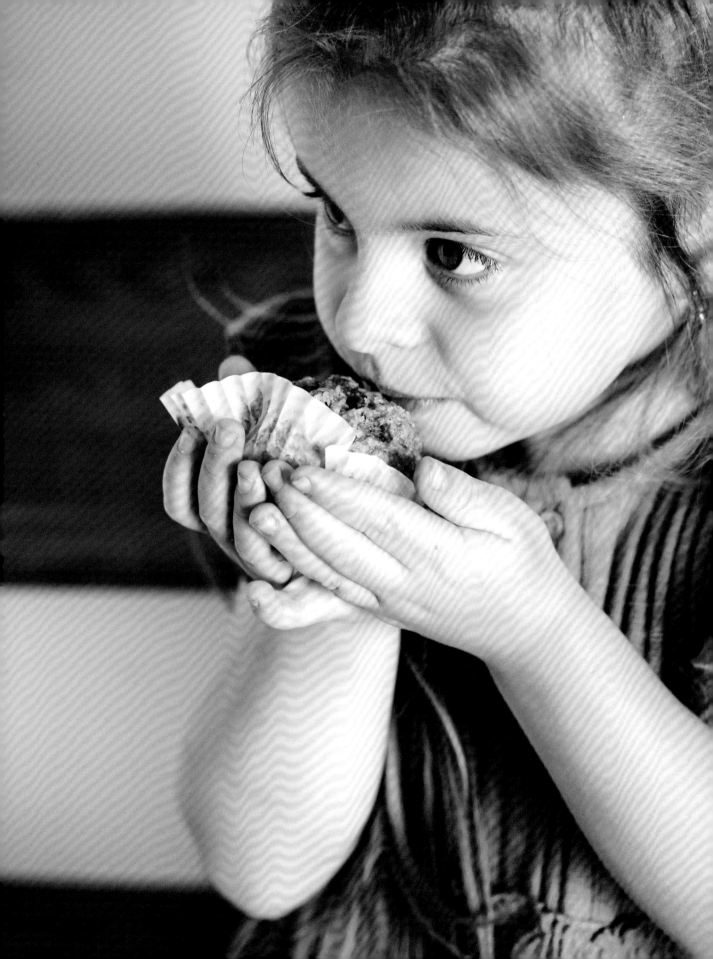

Breakfast

The Mediterranean breakfast is much simpler than ours: tea or coffee with a side of fruit, whole grain crispbreads (such as rye or buckwheat rusks), and perhaps yogurt or cheese drizzled with olive oil. On this side of the Atlantic, we start our days a little differently. This chapter includes delicious Mediterranean-inspired breakfast options that will awaken our taste buds and provide the sustenance we've got used to. Ingredients high in fiber, protein, and fat, such as whole grains, fruit, and nuts, shine in the following recipes, making for a flavorful and energizing way to start the day.

Fig and Olive Oil Granola

Vegetarian • Dairy-free • Gluten-free

Crunchy clusters, chewy figs, and fruity olive oil come together in this nourishing granola. Sprinkle it over yogurt or a smoothie bowl for added texture. It also makes for a great hostess gift, so I like to keep a healthy supply in the freezer. MAKES 6 CUPS (1.5 L)

3 cups (750 mL) certified gluten-free rolled oats

1 cup (250 mL) sliced almonds

1 cup (250 mL) unsweetened shredded coconut

½ cup (125 mL) hemp seeds

3 Tbsp (45 mL) white sesame seeds

½ tsp (2.5 mL) ground cinnamon

¼ tsp (1 mL) sea salt

½ cup (125 mL) honey

¼ cup (60 mL) olive oil

½ tsp (2.5 mL) pure vanilla extract

1½ cups (375 mL) chopped dried figs (see Kitchen Tip)

1. Preheat the oven to 300°F (150°C). Line a baking sheet with parchment paper.

2. In a large bowl, combine the oats, almonds, coconut, hemp seeds, sesame seeds, cinnamon, and salt.

3. To a liquid measuring cup, add the honey, oil, and vanilla. Heat in the microwave for 30 seconds, then whisk to combine.

4. Pour the wet ingredients over the dry ingredients and stir until evenly moistened.

5. Spread the mixture evenly on the prepared baking sheet. Bake for 40 to 45 minutes, stirring halfway through, until the granola is nicely golden brown.

6. Let the granola cool slightly before crumbling. Add the figs and toss until evenly distributed. Serve, or store in an airtight container at room temperature for up to 1 week or in the freezer for up to 3 months.

KITCHEN TIP: If your dried figs are too hard, soak them in hot water for 10 minutes. Drain and pat dry before chopping and adding to the granola.

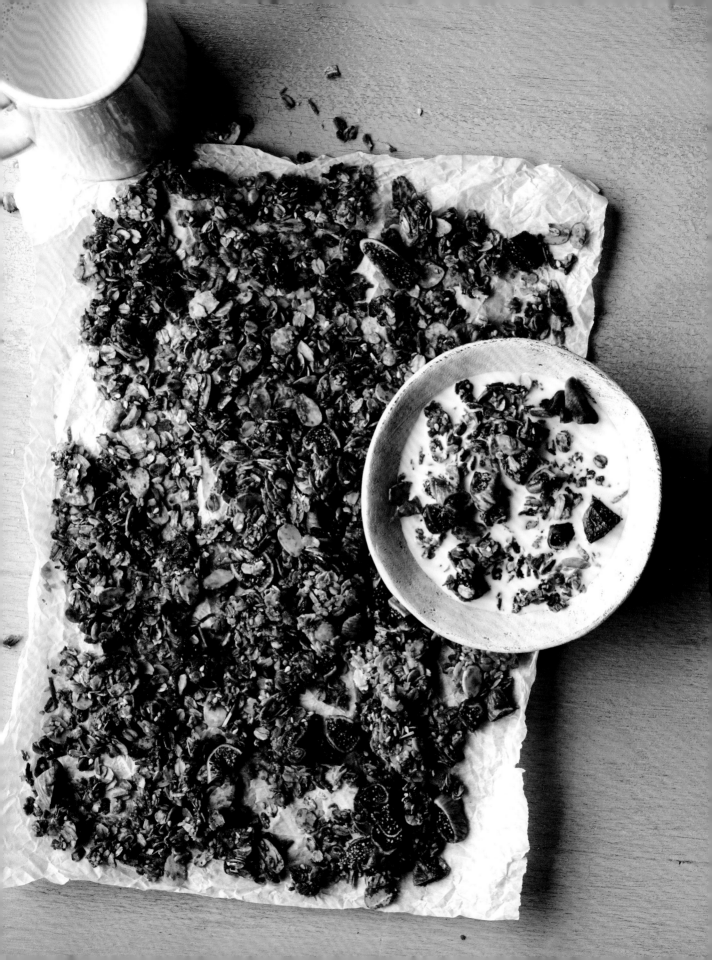

Ricotta-Stuffed French Toast with Blueberry Maple Syrup

Vegetarian • Nut-free

When I was younger, my grandmother would prepare bread and ricotta (both homemade and still warm), topped with a drizzle of olive oil. Some mornings, though, little me would request the "sweet" version, and of course she obliged. Instead of olive oil, a small spoonful of her fig preserves were swirled into the creamy ricotta. This dish is inspired by those flavors and our modern tradition of Saturday brunch. In this version, wild blueberries and maple syrup—two beloved local ingredients—are a natural match and the perfect pairing for the lemon-scented French toast. The natural sweetness of the berries shines through this fruity syrup, which can just as well be drizzled over yogurt, oatmeal, or pancakes. SERVES 4

FOR THE SYRUP

2 cups (500 mL) wild blueberries (fresh or frozen)

⅓ cup (80 mL) pure maple syrup

FOR THE FRENCH TOAST

⅔ cup (160 mL) whole-milk ricotta

½ tsp (2.5 mL) ground cinnamon

Zest of 1 lemon

8 slices of whole grain bread

2 eggs

¼ cup (60 mL) milk

1 tsp (5 mL) pure vanilla extract

1 Tbsp (15 mL) butter

1. **MAKE THE SYRUP** In a small saucepan set over medium heat, bring the blueberries and maple syrup to a boil. Reduce the heat to low and cook for 5 minutes or until the berries are slightly softened. Let cool slightly.

2. **PREPARE THE FRENCH TOAST** In a small bowl, combine the ricotta, cinnamon, and lemon zest. Spread the mixture over 4 slices of bread and cover each with another slice to form sandwiches.

3. In a shallow bowl, whisk together the eggs, milk, and vanilla.

4. Heat a 12-inch (30 cm) non-stick skillet over medium heat and lightly grease the pan with the butter.

5. While the skillet is heating, dip the sandwiches in the egg mixture, coating them well. In batches so as not to overcrowd, cook the French toast in the hot skillet until golden brown, about 3 minutes per side. Set aside on a plate, covered with foil, until all the sandwiches are cooked.

6. Slice the French toast sandwiches in half diagonally. Serve with the blueberry maple syrup.

KITCHEN TIP: Frozen fruit is just as nutritious as fresh, making it an excellent option, especially out of season.

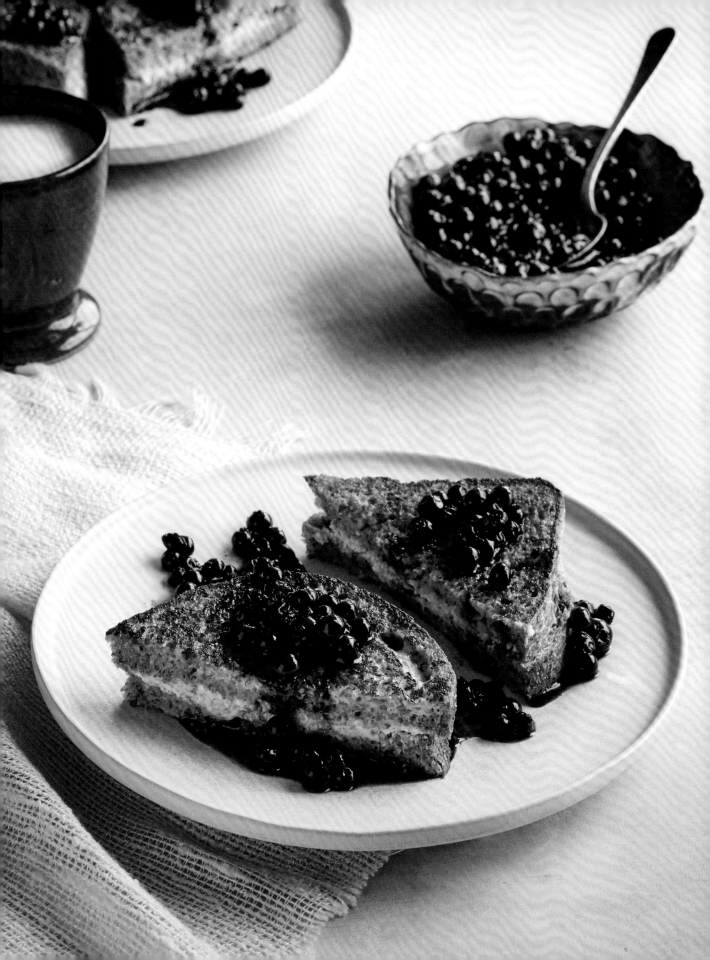

Walnut Zucchini Muffins

Vegetarian • Dairy-free

Nutty, not too sweet, and perfectly moist thanks to the grated zucchini, these muffins are a go-to in my home. The secret to a good muffin? Using a light hand and not over-mixing. I like to use a fork in the final combining stages, to use as few strokes as possible. MAKES 9 MUFFINS

1 cup (250 mL) raw walnuts (see Nutrition Note)

1 cup (250 mL) quick-cooking oats

1 cup (250 mL) all-purpose flour

3 Tbsp (45 mL) ground flaxseed

1 tsp (5 mL) ground cinnamon

1 tsp (5 mL) baking powder

½ tsp (2.5 mL) baking soda

¼ tsp (1 mL) salt

¼ cup (60 mL) olive or vegetable oil

½ cup (125 mL) honey

2 large eggs

1 tsp (5 mL) pure vanilla extract

1 cup (250 mL) grated zucchini

2 Tbsp (30 mL) turbinado sugar

1. Preheat the oven to 375°F (190°C). Grease a standard-size 9-cup muffin tin.

2. Place the walnuts on a baking sheet and bake for 5 minutes or until fragrant. Let the nuts cool slightly, then finely chop.

3. In a large bowl, combine the oats, flour, flaxseed, cinnamon, baking powder, baking soda, and salt.

4. In a small bowl, whisk together the oil, honey, eggs, and vanilla.

5. Pour the liquid ingredients over the dry ingredients and mix to combine. Stir in the walnuts and zucchini.

6. Using an ice cream scoop, divide the batter evenly among the muffin cups. Top each with a sprinkling of sugar.

7. Bake for 18 to 20 minutes, until the tops of the muffins are golden and spring back slightly to the touch.

8. Let cool in the tin for 10 minutes before unmolding. Serve warm. Any leftovers can be stored in an airtight container in the freezer for up to 3 months.

NUTRITION NOTE: Ever notice how walnuts look like tiny brains? What a coincidence, given that walnuts are high in plant-based omega-3 fatty acids, important nutrients for brain growth and health.

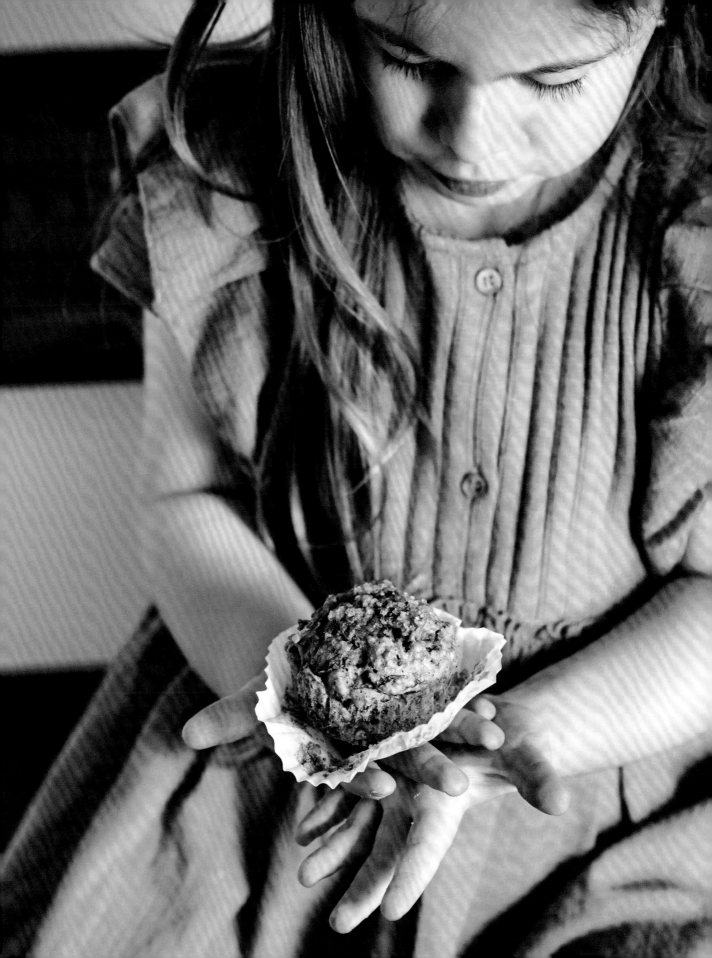

Cherry, Cacao, and Olive Oil Smoothie

Vegan • Vegetarian • Dairy-free • Gluten-free

This smoothie is my homage to the old Mediterranean ritual of starting the day with a swig of liquid gold. The natural fruitiness of quality extra virgin olive oil is the perfect complement to the cherries in this smoothie, which are rounded out with a touch of cacao powder for warmth and richness. The ingredients in this recipe not only make for a refreshing drink but also provide the necessary nutrients for any morning meal. Oat milk stands out from other plant-based drinks for its fiber content, while almond butter adds a dose of healthy fat—key elements to keep hunger and energy levels on an even keel all morning. SERVES 2

1½ cups (375 mL) unsweetened oat milk

2 cups (500 mL) frozen cherries

1 Tbsp (15 mL) almond butter

2 tsp (10 mL) raw cacao powder

2 tsp (10 mL) extra virgin olive oil

1 large handful baby spinach

Pinch of ground cinnamon

2 Tbsp (30 mL) plant-based vanilla protein powder (optional)

1. Place all the ingredients in a blender, and blend until smooth.

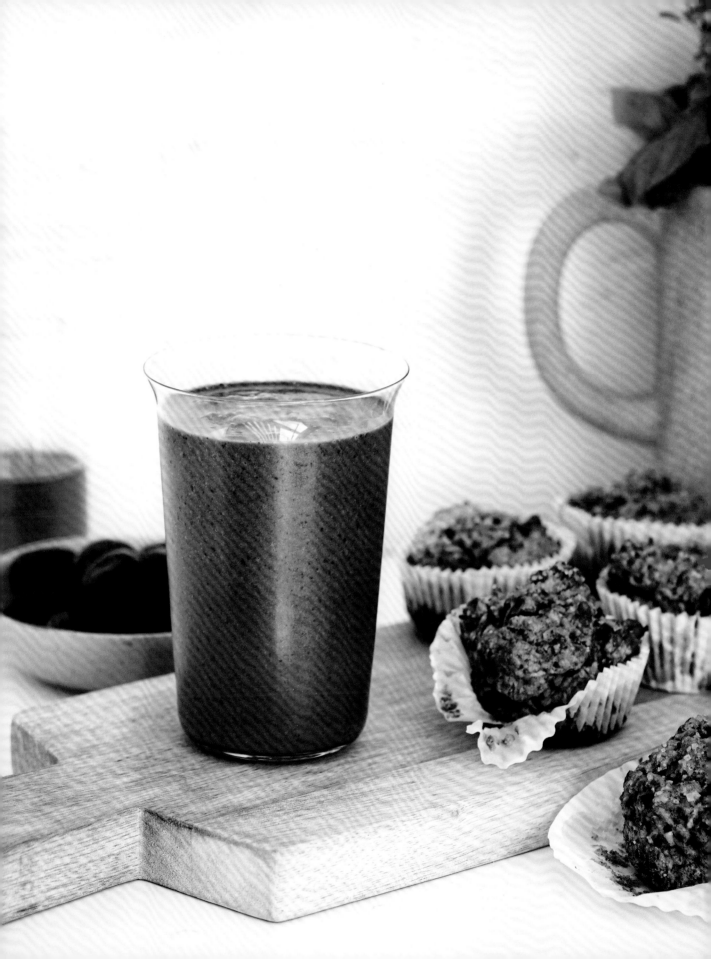

Egg, Lima Bean, and Feta Breakfast Skillet

Vegetarian • Gluten-free • Nut-free

This dish is a cross between the traditional Greek dish *gigantes plaki* and the Italian Eggs in Purgatory. The result is a comforting and filling meal, fit for a leisurely brunch or even a speedy weeknight dinner. Lima beans (also known as butter beans) have a buttery flesh and delicate flavor that works well in many soups, stews, and salads. They also clock in at 13 grams of protein per cup (250 mL), making them a budget-friendly, plant-based protein source that is worth a regular spot in your grocery cart. SERVES 4

2 Tbsp (30 mL) olive oil

1 onion, chopped

1 celery stalk, sliced

2 garlic cloves, halved

1 can (19 oz/540 mL) lima beans,
   drained and rinsed (see Kitchen Tip)

1 can (14 oz/398 mL) diced tomatoes

½ cup (125 mL) water

1 tsp (5 mL) honey

½ tsp (2.5 mL) dried oregano

1 bay leaf

Pinch of ground cinnamon

Salt and pepper

4 eggs

¼ cup (60 mL) crumbled feta

4 slices of crusty sourdough bread
   (gluten-free if necessary),
   to serve

1. Preheat the oven to 350°F (180°C).

2. Heat the olive oil in a 12-inch (30 cm) ovenproof skillet set over medium heat. Add the onion, celery, and garlic, and sauté for 5 minutes.

3. Add the beans, tomatoes, water, honey, oregano, bay leaf, and cinnamon. Season with salt and pepper. Bring to a simmer and cook for 10 minutes, then remove from the heat.

4. Crack the eggs directly into the sauce, then transfer to the oven. Bake for 8 to 10 minutes, until the egg whites are set but the yolks are still runny. Remove from the oven, top with the feta, and serve with crusty bread.

KITCHEN TIP: Have dried lima beans at home? See "Cooking with Dried Pulses," page 39, to learn how to prep them to use in this recipe. Measure 2 cups (500 mL) cooked beans and proceed with this recipe.

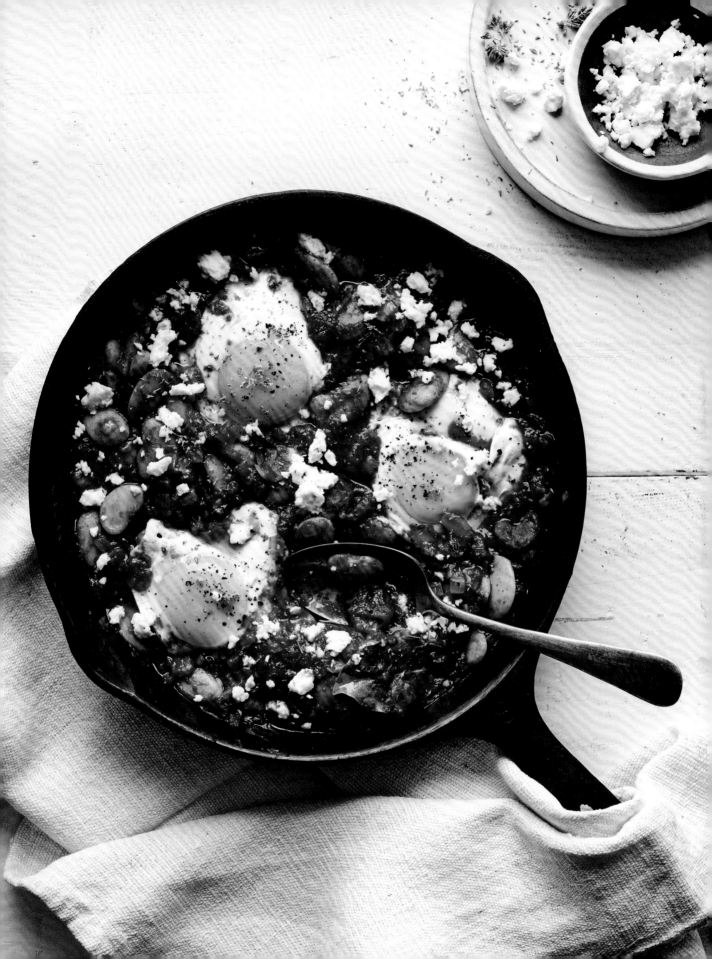

Bruschetta-Style Pea and Avocado Toast

Vegan • Vegetarian • Dairy-free • Nut-free

The famous avocado toast gets a makeover here thanks to the addition of peas. They not only impart a freshness to the dish but also provide a satisfying dose of fiber and protein, making this a complete breakfast option. The bright and acidic bruschetta topping brings it all together, for a delicious wake-up call. SERVES 2

1 cup (250 mL) quartered grape tomatoes

1 shallot, minced

¼ cup (60 mL) coarsely chopped fresh basil

2 Tbsp (30 mL) extra virgin olive oil

2 tsp (10 mL) balsamic vinegar

Salt and pepper

1 cup (250 mL) frozen green peas

1 ripe avocado, pitted, peeled, and coarsely chopped

Juice of ½ lemon

2 slices of crusty sourdough bread (see Kitchen Tip)

1 garlic clove, halved

1. In a small bowl, combine the tomatoes, shallot, basil, oil, vinegar, and salt and pepper to taste. Set this bruschetta mixture aside.

2. In a small saucepan, bring salted water to a boil. Add the green peas and cook for 5 minutes. Drain and transfer to a bowl.

3. Mash the peas with a fork. Add the avocado, lemon juice, and more salt and pepper to taste. Mix until the ingredients are combined but the texture is still chunky.

4. Toast the bread. Rub the warm toast with the cut sides of the garlic clove. Spread the pea and avocado mash on the bread, then top with the bruschetta mixture.

KITCHEN TIP: Head to your local bakery and explore its sourdough options. Because sourdough is fermented, it offers a flavor that many people find more satisfying than traditional grocery store options. Interestingly, the unique fermentation optimizes the nutrition value and may make the bread easier to digest. Look for options made with whole grain flours, and have your loaf sliced for easy access to bakery-style bread once it's in the freezer. It will keep in the freezer for up to 3 months.

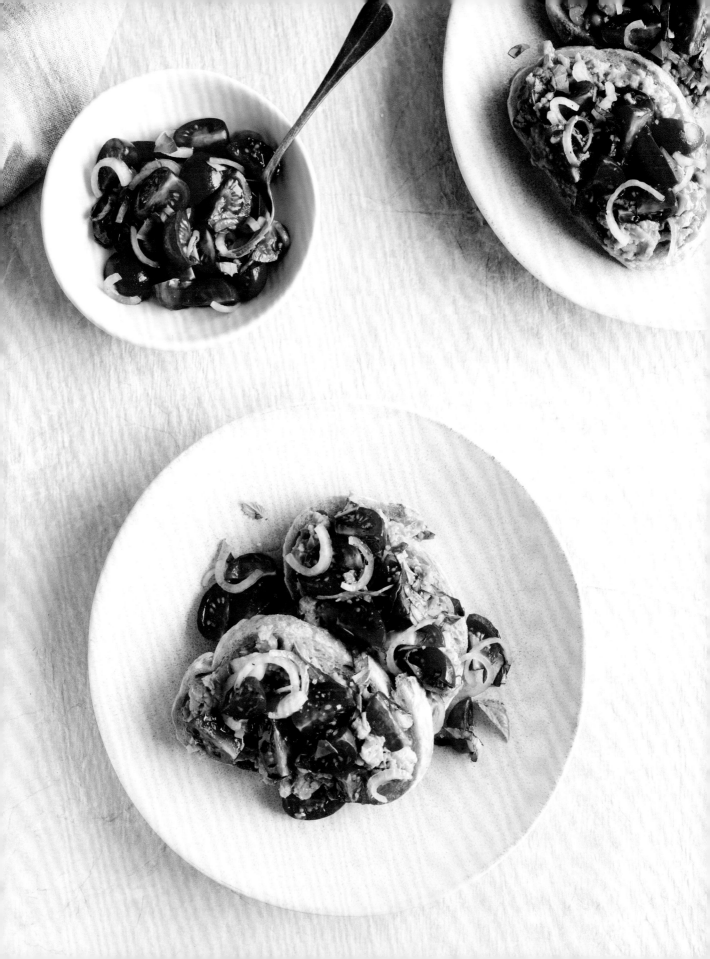

Egg and Halloumi Breakfast Plate

Vegetarian • Gluten-free • Nut-free

This recipe brings me back to the "eggs in a hole" I came to love as a child. But instead of bread, this grown-up version cracks the egg onto a slice of grilled halloumi! This recipe highlights two key Mediterranean ingredients we tend to shy away from at breakfast time: vegetables and spices. Yet fragrant za'atar, wilted spinach, and bursting tomatoes make this dish a flavorful and colorful way to start the day. SERVES 2

1 tsp (5 mL) olive oil

½ onion, chopped

1 cup (250 mL) halved grape tomatoes

1 cup (250 mL) packed baby spinach

Salt and pepper

Two ½-inch-thick (1.2 cm) slices halloumi

2 eggs

1 tsp (5 mL) za'atar, store-bought or homemade (page 245) (see Kitchen Tip)

2 Tbsp (30 mL) water

1. Heat the olive oil in a 10-inch (25 cm) non-stick skillet set over medium-low heat. Add the onion and sauté for 2 minutes. Add the tomatoes and spinach, then season with salt and pepper. Cook for 1 minute or until the spinach has wilted and the tomatoes have slightly softened. Transfer to a plate.

2. In the same skillet, sear the halloumi on one side until golden brown. Flip the halloumi and crack one egg onto each slice of cheese. Sprinkle the eggs with the za'atar.

3. As the egg whites begin to harden, add a splash of water to the outer rim of the pan to create steam, then quickly cover with a lid. Cook until the egg whites are firm but the yolks are still runny, about 2 minutes. Serve alongside the vegetables.

KITCHEN TIP: Za'atar is a fragrant blend of oregano, thyme, sumac, and sesame. With its herbaceous notes and slight acidity, this blend goes well with a variety of foods. You can find it in the spice section of your grocery store or make your own (page 245).

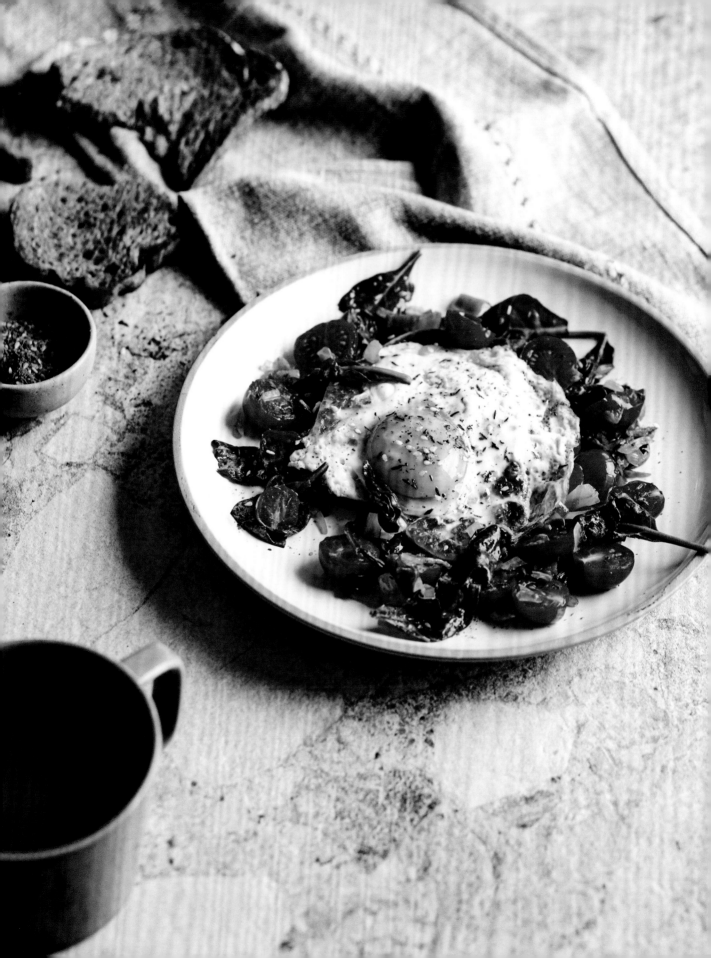

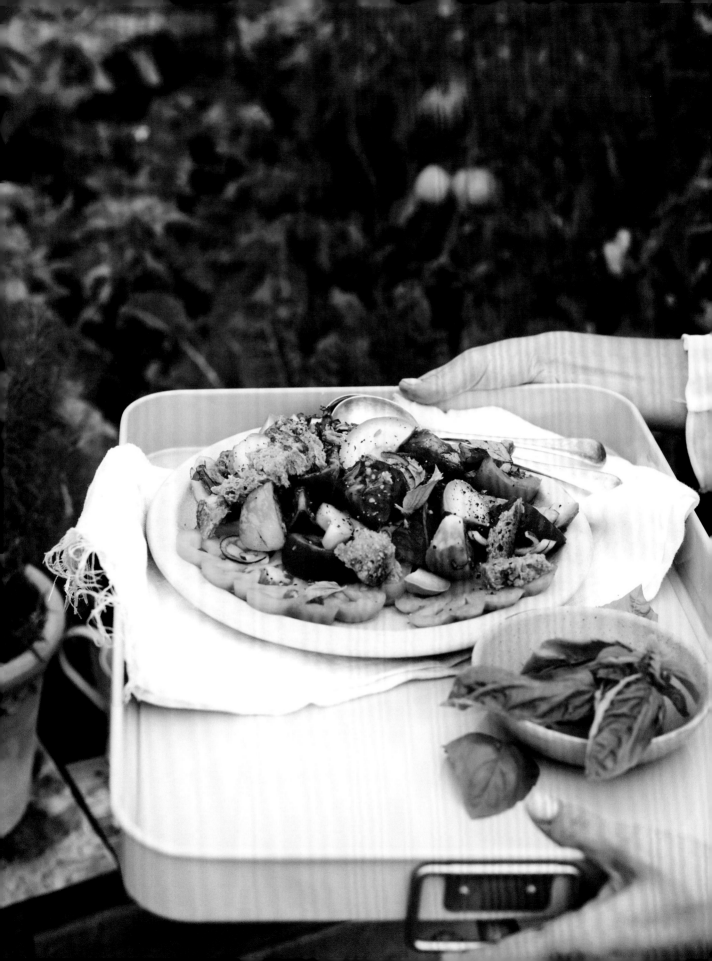

Soups and Salads

Some of the dishes that immediately come to mind when we think of the Mediterranean are soups and salads, and it's no wonder. Soups and salads are a simple way to transform bountiful harvests into nourishing, budget-friendly dishes that can feed a family. You'll be sure to find plenty of vegetables, whole grains (like my favorite, farro), and pulses in the following recipes, in keeping with the Mediterranean diet principles of seasonality, frugality, and plant-forward cooking. They can serve as the plant-forward first course at your next dinner party or for everyday meals with your family.

Creamy Tuscan Soup with Sausage, White Beans, and Kale

Dairy-free • Gluten-free • Nut-free

White beans are the secret to the creamy texture of this soup. When puréed, they add that luscious creaminess—without the cream—along with a dose of both fiber and protein. I tend to rely on white beans for this in my soups, which is why I keep cans of them in my pantry, at the ready. SERVES 6 TO 8

1 lb (450 g) mild Italian sausage, casings removed

1 Tbsp (15 mL) olive oil

1 onion, finely chopped

1 celery stalk, finely sliced

2 cups (500 mL) chopped leeks

3 garlic cloves, minced

2 cups (500 mL) peeled and diced yellow or Yukon Gold potatoes

1 can (19 oz/540 mL) cannellini beans, drained and rinsed (see Kitchen Tip)

6 cups (1.5 L) no-salt-added chicken broth

1 large sprig of rosemary

Salt and pepper

4 cups (1 L) thinly sliced kale

1. In a large pot set over medium heat, cook the sausage for 10 minutes, breaking up the meat into small pieces using a fork or wooden spoon. Transfer to a bowl.

2. In the same pan set over medium heat, cook the olive oil, onion, celery, leeks, and garlic for 5 minutes. Add the potatoes and beans, then the broth and rosemary. Season with salt and pepper, then bring to a boil.

3. Reduce the heat to medium-low and simmer for 15 minutes or until the potatoes are cooked through. Remove the rosemary.

4. Transfer 3 cups (750 mL) of the soup to a blender and purée until smooth. Return to the saucepan and stir to combine.

5. Add the sausage and kale to the soup, then cook for 5 to 10 minutes, to soften the kale. Season with more salt and pepper, and serve. Any leftovers can be stored in an airtight container in the refrigerator for up to 4 days or in the freezer for up to 3 months.

KITCHEN TIP: Have dried white beans at home? See "Cooking with Dried Pulses," page 39, to learn how to prep them to use in this recipe. Measure 2 cups (500 mL) cooked beans and proceed with this recipe.

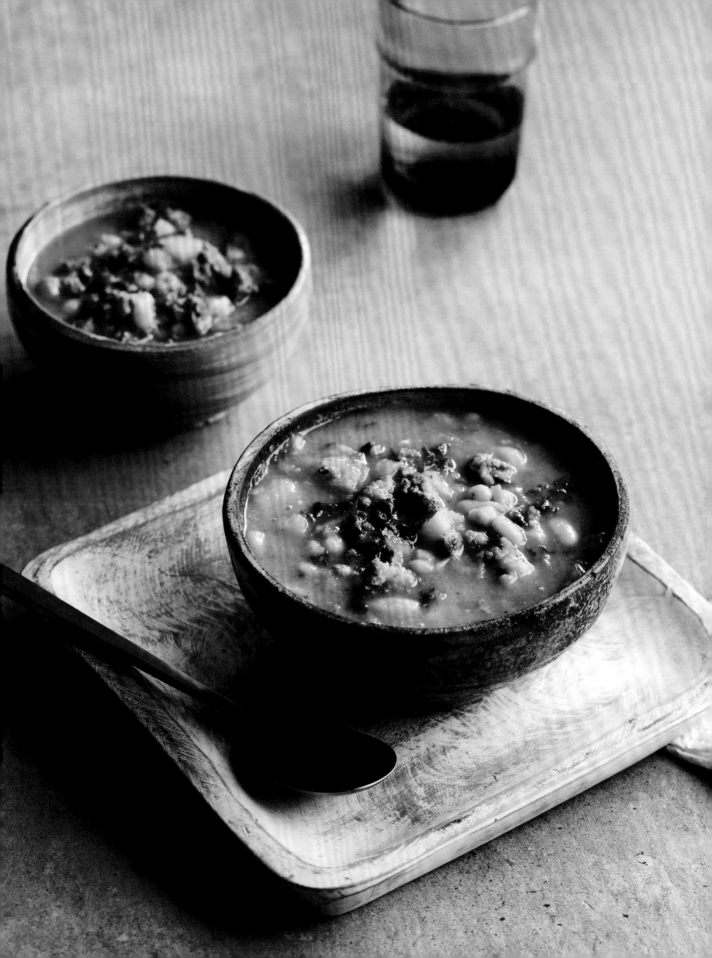

Farro e Fagioli

Vegetarian • Nut-free

This hearty dish of farro and beans is the essence of the Mediterranean diet. Simple, humble ingredients come together to create a delicious meal for a family, made complete thanks to the high-fiber farro and protein-rich beans. The parmesan rind makes all the difference in simple dishes like this one, so be sure not to skip it. It adds richness and umami for depth of flavor. SERVES 4 TO 6

2 Tbsp (30 mL) olive oil

2 cups (500 mL) finely chopped onion

2 garlic cloves, halved

½ tsp (2.5 mL) crushed chili flakes

1 cup (250 mL) farro, rinsed

1 can (19 oz/540 mL) romano beans, drained and rinsed

4 cups (1 L) low-sodium vegetable broth

3 cups (750 mL) water

¾ cup (180 mL) canned diced tomatoes

10 basil leaves, coarsely torn

1 bay leaf

1 Parmigiano Reggiano rind (about 2 inches/5 cm long) (see Kitchen Tip)

Salt and pepper

1. Heat the olive oil in a large pot set over medium heat. Add the onion, garlic, and chili flakes. Cook until softened, about 4 minutes, stirring frequently and taking care not to brown the vegetables. Add the farro, stir to coat the grains, and cook for 3 minutes.

2. Add the beans, broth, water, tomatoes, basil, bay leaf, and parmesan rind. Season with salt and pepper. Bring to a boil, then reduce the heat to medium-low and let simmer, uncovered, for 30 minutes or until the farro is tender but still has a bit of chew to it. Remove the bay leaf and rind. Season with more salt and pepper, and serve. Any leftovers can be stored in an airtight container in the refrigerator for up to 4 days or in the freezer for up to 3 months.

KITCHEN TIP: Buy your Parmigiano Reggiano in a block, rather than grated. This way you can grate your cheese fresh as needed, but also keep the rind. I keep a bag of the rinds in the freezer, always adding a piece when preparing a soup, for depth of flavor.

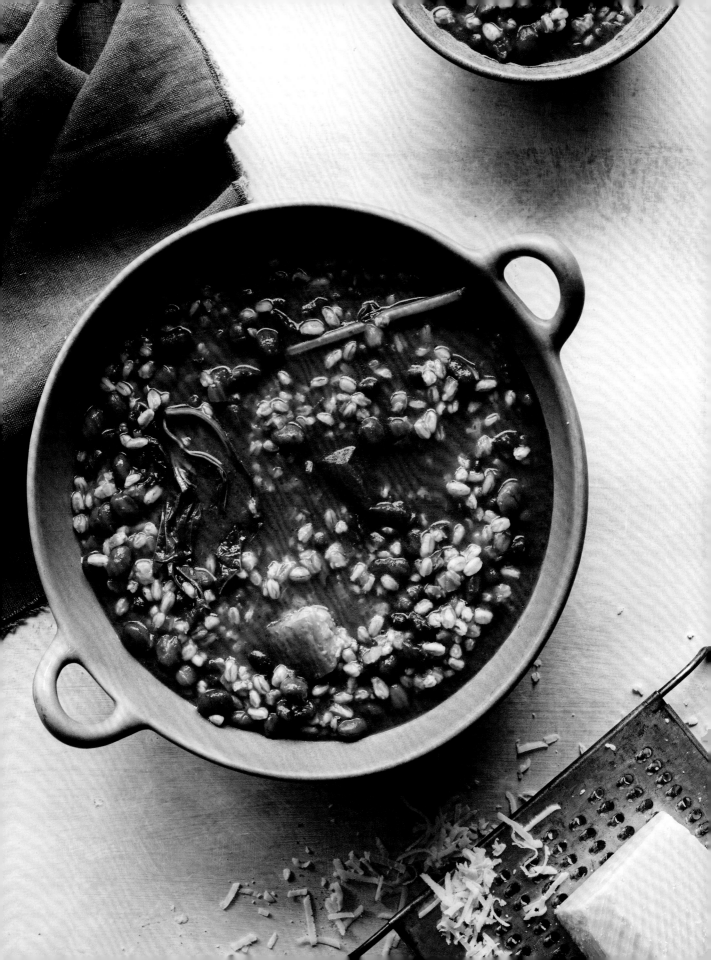

Roasted Tomato and Lentil Soup with Halloumi Croutons

Vegetarian • Gluten-free • Nut-free

Red lentils turn this classic soup into a complete meal, packing protein and fiber in every very velvety spoonful. The best part? The halloumi "croutons" you will enjoy fishing out with every bite. It's like a grilled cheese and tomato soup. SERVES 4 TO 6

2 lb (1 kg) Roma tomatoes (about 10 to 12), halved lengthwise

4 garlic cloves, crushed

4 Tbsp (60 mL) olive oil, divided

Salt and pepper

1 cup (250 mL) ½-inch (1.2 cm) cubed halloumi

2 cups (500 mL) chopped onion

2 Tbsp (30 mL) tomato paste

1 cup (250 mL) dried red lentils (see Kitchen Tip)

6 cups (1.5 L) vegetable broth

1 cup (250 mL) packed fresh basil, plus more to garnish

1. Preheat the oven to 400°F (200°C). Line a baking sheet with parchment paper.

2. Place the tomatoes and garlic on the prepared baking sheet. Drizzle with 3 Tbsp (45 mL) oil and toss to evenly coat the vegetables. Season with salt and pepper. Place in the oven and roast for 35 to 40 minutes, stirring halfway through, or until the tomatoes caramelize. Set aside.

3. In a 10-inch (25 cm) non-stick skillet set over medium-high heat, sear the halloumi cubes until golden brown on all sides. Set aside.

4. Heat the remaining 1 Tbsp (15 mL) oil in a large pot set over medium-high heat. Add the onion and tomato paste, stir to combine, and cook until softened, about 7 minutes. Add the lentils, then the broth, basil, and roasted tomatoes. Bring to a boil, then reduce the heat to medium and simmer for 15 to 20 minutes, until the lentils are tender. Remove from the heat.

5. Using a hand blender, purée the soup until smooth. Season with salt and pepper. Serve the soup hot, garnished with the seared halloumi cubes and basil. Store the soup in an airtight container in the refrigerator for up to 4 days or in the freezer for up to 3 months.

KITCHEN TIP: Unlike other pulses, dried lentils do not need to be soaked before cooking. And since they cook up fast, I lean on dried rather than canned lentils as my pantry staple. For all other pulses, I like to keep a combination of dried and canned options, alternating between them depending on how pressed I am for time. See page 39 for more on cooking with dried pulses.

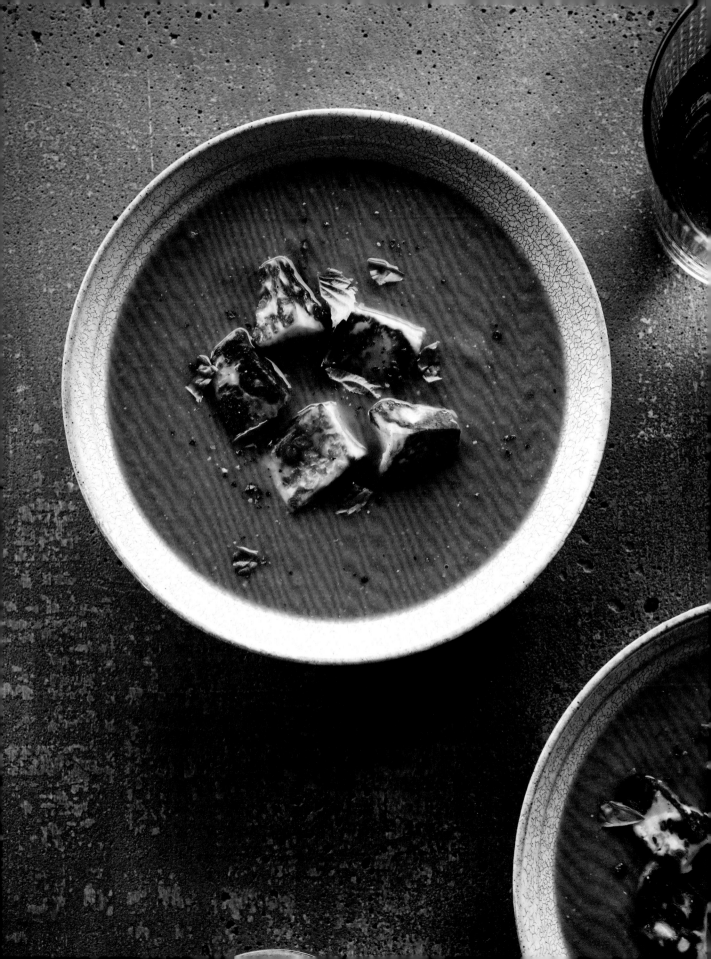

Panzanella with Avocado

Vegan • Vegetarian • Dairy-free • Nut-free

The panzanella was born of necessity, giving a second life to stale bread that otherwise would be thrown away. The basics of a panzanella are in-season tomatoes, crunchy cucumbers, sharp red onion, and, of course, bread, tossed in quality olive oil and a splash of red wine vinegar. The bread in this salad acts as a flavor magnet, soaking up the fresh tomato juices and seasoned olive oil. Beyond this, the dish is quite flexible. This version includes sliced avocado, for a touch of creaminess, which pairs beautifully with this bright, acidic salad. Avocado isn't a traditional Mediterranean ingredient, but one I've come to love. Mostly known for its healthy fat content, avocado is also high in fiber and potassium, a key nutrient we struggle to get enough of in our diet. This means that this salad not only comes packed with flavor but is bursting with nourishing ingredients, making it the ideal summer side dish to pair with a simple grilled fish or to include in your next al fresco spread. SERVES 4

4 slices of crusty bread or half of a baguette (preferably day-old)

2 lb (1 kg) heirloom tomatoes, cut into wedges

1 cucumber, halved lengthwise and sliced

½ cup (125 mL) coarsely chopped fresh basil, plus more to garnish

½ red onion, thinly sliced

1 garlic clove, halved

¼ cup (60 mL) extra virgin olive oil

2 Tbsp (30 mL) quality red wine vinegar

Salt and pepper

1 ripe but firm avocado, pitted, peeled, and sliced

1. Preheat the oven to 325°F (165°C). Line a baking sheet with parchment paper.

2. Tear the bread into 2-inch (5 cm) pieces and spread evenly on the baking sheet. Bake for 20 to 25 minutes, until dry and slightly golden. Cool completely.

3. In a large bowl, toss together the toasted bread, tomatoes, cucumber, basil, onion, garlic, oil, and vinegar. Season with salt and pepper. Let the salad rest for 10 minutes, to allow the bread to soak up the juices. Remove the garlic.

4. Transfer to a serving platter and top with the avocado. Garnish with the basil and serve.

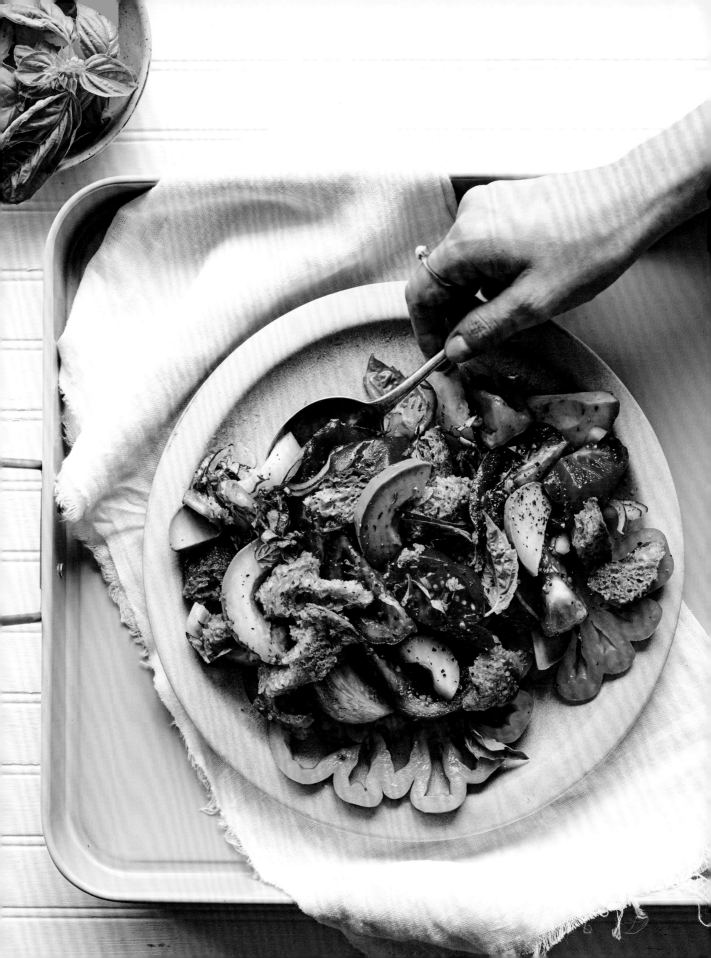

Warm Mushroom, Farro, and Radicchio Salad

Vegetarian • Nut-free

This salad of bitter radicchio, creamy parmesan, nutty farro, and earthy mushrooms will be your go-to in colder months. If you are unfamiliar with farro, I hope this recipe makes you take the plunge and try it. Farro is an ancient grain and a relative to wheat, but providing more protein, fiber, and B vitamins. It has a unique chewy texture and nutty flavor, which, combined with its nutritional profile, make it a wonderful way to turn salads into filling and satisfying dishes. This recipe makes for a lovely appetizer or side dish, but you can also top it with soft-boiled eggs for a balanced dinner option. SERVES 4

½ cup (125 mL) farro, rinsed

2 Tbsp (30 mL) olive oil, divided

1 package (8 oz/227 g) cremini mushrooms, sliced

2 garlic cloves, halved

2 sprigs of thyme

2 Tbsp (30 mL) balsamic vinegar, divided

½ head radicchio, sliced

Salt and pepper

⅓ cup (80 mL) Parmigiano Reggiano shavings

1. In a saucepan, bring salted water to a boil. Add the farro and cook for 20 to 30 minutes, until al dente. Drain and set aside.

2. In a 10-inch (25 cm) non-stick skillet set over medium, heat 1 Tbsp (15 mL) oil. Add the mushrooms, garlic, and thyme, and sauté for 6 minutes, or until the mushrooms have softened.

3. Add 1 Tbsp (15 mL) vinegar and reduce, 1 minute. Remove the pan from the heat. Remove the garlic cloves and thyme stems, and reserve.

4. In a bowl, combine the cooked farro, radicchio, the remaining 1 Tbsp (15 mL) oil, and the remaining 1 Tbsp (15 mL) vinegar. Toss, then season with salt and pepper.

5. Transfer the farro and radicchio salad to a serving platter. Top with the warm mushrooms and parmesan shavings.

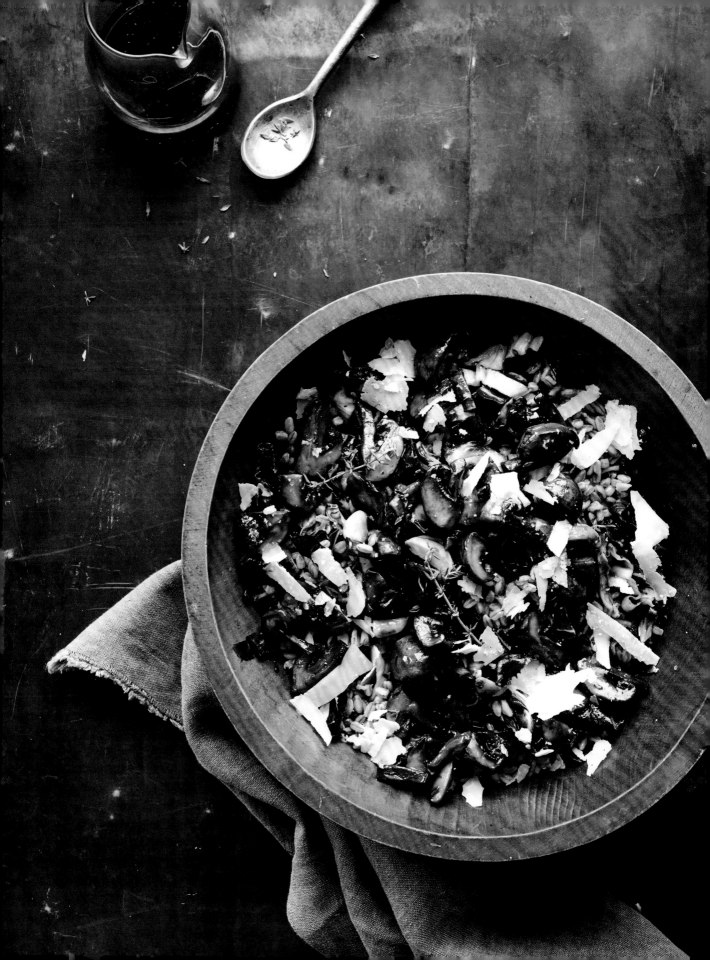

Tuna, Egg, and Potato Salad

Vegetarian • Dairy-free • Gluten-free • Nut-free

I consider this salad a simplified version of the classic Niçoise. It pairs pantry staple ingredients like potatoes and canned tuna with fresh tomatoes, lettuce, and boiled eggs, plus a simple olive oil dressing. So, although it comes together simply, it eats like a meal with its filling, protein-rich ingredients. This colorful salad would make for a beautiful dish for a picnic in the park or an energizing lunch prepped ahead of a busy workweek. SERVES 4

4 eggs

4 Yukon Gold potatoes, peeled and cut into wedges

3 Tbsp (45 mL) extra virgin olive oil, divided

Salt and pepper

4 Roma tomatoes, quartered

2 green onions, sliced

¼ cup (60 mL) finely chopped fresh flat-leaf parsley

4 cups (1 L) packed chopped romaine lettuce

Juice of ½ lemon

1 jar (6.7 oz/190 g) tuna filets, drained (see Kitchen Tip)

1. Place the eggs in a small saucepan, cover with cold water, and bring to a boil. Once boiling, remove from the heat, cover with a lid, and let stand 12 minutes. Drain and peel the eggs, then cut them in half lengthwise.

2. Place the potatoes in a saucepan, cover with cold, salted water, and bring to a boil. Cook for 15 minutes or until fork-tender. Drain the potatoes and transfer to a large bowl. While they are still hot, drizzle with 1 Tbsp (15 mL) oil and season with salt and pepper. Toss and let cool slightly.

3. Add the tomatoes, green onions, and parsley, followed by the lettuce, the remaining 2 Tbsp (30 mL) olive oil, lemon juice, and salt and pepper to taste. Toss and top with the boiled eggs and tuna filets.

KITCHEN TIP: Jarred tuna, with its longer, meatier filets, can be found at the grocery store next to its canned counterpart. That said, a can of tuna can be used instead for this recipe, if you like.

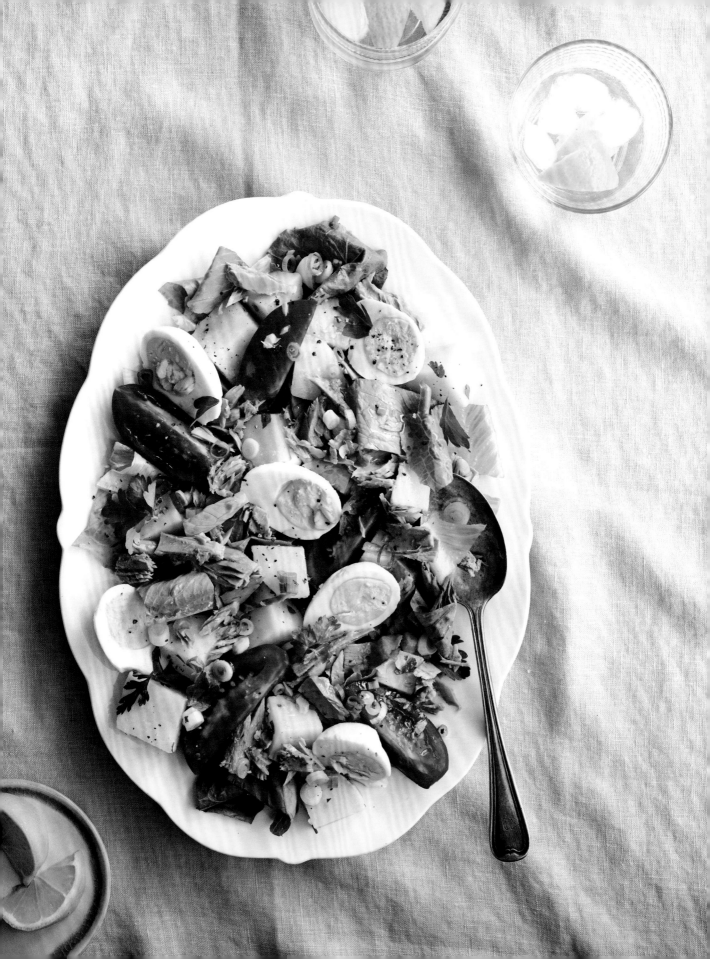

Fennel and Orange Salad

Vegan · Vegetarian · Dairy-free · Gluten-free · Nut-free

This classic salad is a celebration of simplicity and seasonality—pillars of the Mediterranean cooking style. It also packs a punch of vitamin C and fiber, thanks to its two star ingredients. The combination of crisp fennel, salty olives, sharp onion, and sweet oranges makes for an addictive salad that will turn any fennel doubter into a fennel lover. This dish makes a great salad course, and is also perfect served with the Baked Salmon with Gremolata Crust (page 182). To double up on the fennel flavor, prepare this recipe using my Olives with Fennel and Chili (page 114). SERVES 4 TO 6

2 fennel bulbs with fronds, halved lengthwise (see Kitchen Tip)

4 blood oranges (or Cara Cara), peeled and segmented

½ red onion, thinly sliced

⅓ cup (80 mL) salt-cured black olives, pitted

3 Tbsp (45 mL) extra virgin olive oil

1 Tbsp (15 mL) white wine vinegar

Juice collected from the orange prep (optional)

Salt and pepper

1. Tear the fennel fronds off the stalk and set them aside for the garnish. Using a sharp knife, make a V-shaped incision in the heart of the fennel bulb, removing the tough center while keeping the bulb intact. Thinly slice the fennel using a mandoline (set at ¼ inch/6 mm) or a knife.

2. Place the sliced fennel, orange segments, onion, and olives in a large bowl.

3. In a small bowl, whisk together the oil, vinegar, and any orange juice collected during the prep. Pour the dressing over the fennel and toss to evenly coat. Season with salt and pepper.

4. Transfer to a serving platter, and garnish with the reserved fennel fronds.

KITCHEN TIP: Look for fennel with brightly colored fronds and that feels heavy for its size, without any bruising. To store, wrap in a clean kitchen towel and tuck into a sealed bag. Store in the refrigerator for up to 1 week.

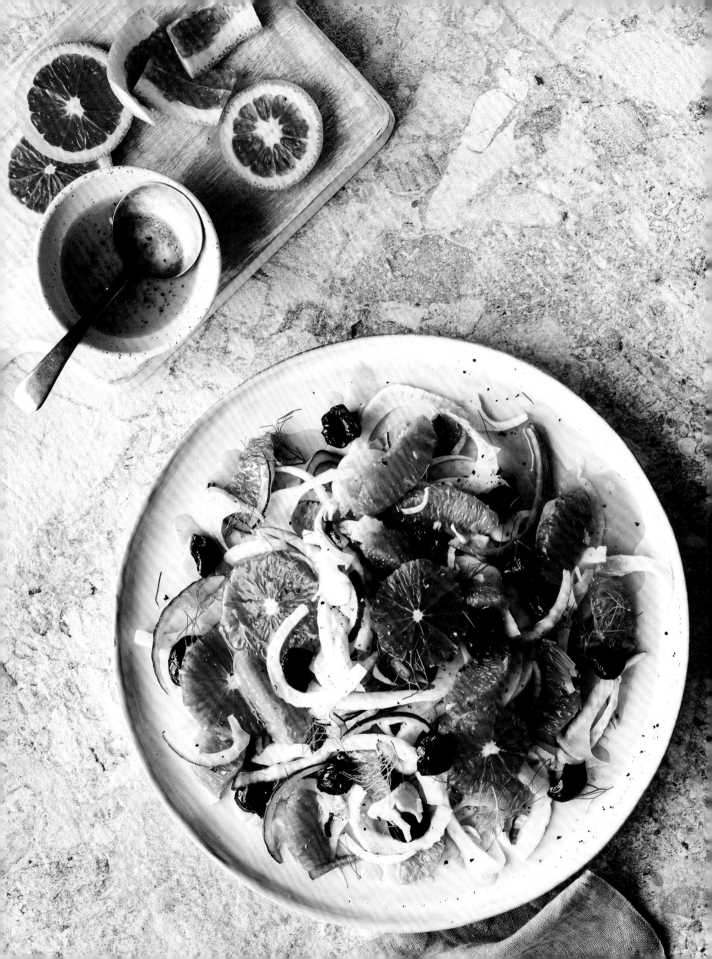

Lentil Tabbouleh

Vegan • Vegetarian • Dairy-free • Gluten-free • Nut-free

In this recipe, hearty lentils replace the traditional bulgur, adding a healthy dose of plant protein, fiber, extra protein, and key nutrients like potassium, folate, and iron. Lentils are a common Mediterranean ingredient, but did you know that *Canada* is the world's leading producer? All the more reason to embrace this tiny-but-mighty pulse in your every day. As a standalone meal, I like to serve this tabbouleh with crisp romaine boats. It can also be served as a side dish, with a simple grilled fish, for example. SERVES 4

1 cup (250 mL) French (Puy) lentils

1 bunch of flat-leaf parsley, finely chopped (see Kitchen Tip)

1 cup (250 mL) finely chopped fresh mint

4 shallots, minced

1 cup (250 mL) finely diced Roma tomatoes

1 cup (250 mL) finely diced cucumber

1 garlic clove, finely chopped

Juice of ½ lemon

3 Tbsp (45 mL) extra virgin olive oil

1 Tbsp (15 mL) za'atar, store-bought or homemade (page 245)

Salt and pepper

10 romaine lettuce leaves (optional)

1. In a large saucepan, bring salted water to a boil. Add the lentils and cook until tender, about 20 minutes. Drain and cool to room temperature.

2. In a large bowl, mix together the lentils, parsley, mint, shallots, tomatoes, cucumber, garlic, lemon juice, oil, za'atar, and salt and pepper to taste. Serve over lettuce leaves.

KITCHEN TIP: The secret to storing fresh herbs? Give them the flower treatment. Purchase fresh herbs like parsley or mint in bunches when possible, trim the stems, and place the bunch in a container with a ½ inch (1.2 cm) of water. Keep in the refrigerator, covered with a plastic resealable bag, and trim freshly as needed. Twice weekly, change the water and trim the stems to freshen them.

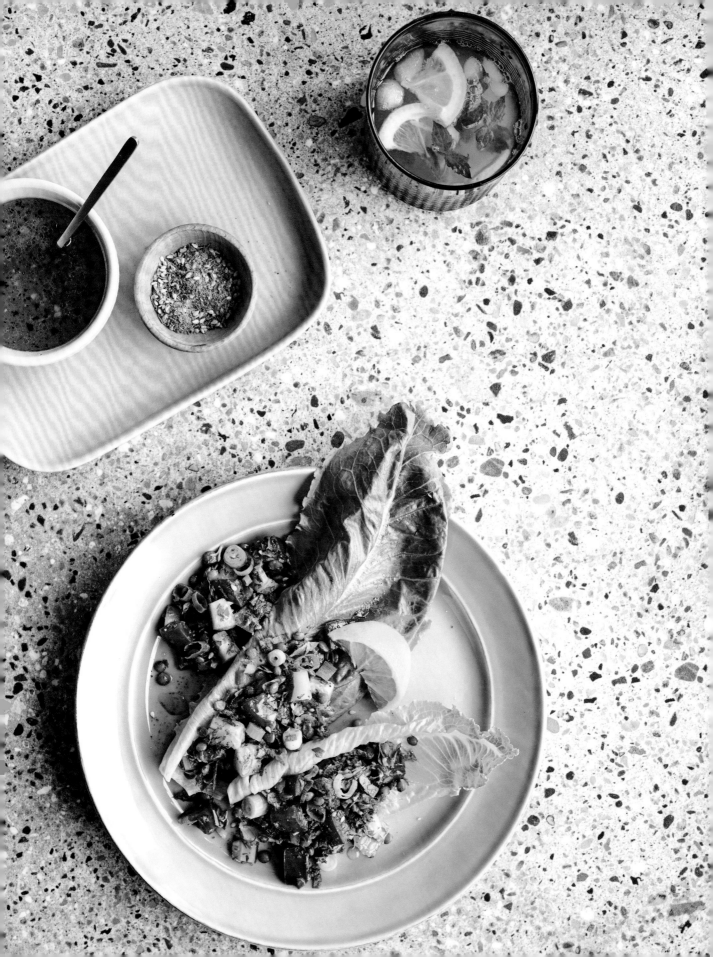

Endive and Persimmon Salad

Vegetarian • Dairy-free • Gluten-free

Mediterranean persimmons (or as I grew up calling them, cachi) are in season in the late fall and early winter, a season so short-lived, you have to catch them when you can and make the most of them. Its beautiful orange flesh is ripe with antioxidant beta-carotene, a nutrient the body transforms into vitamin A, needed for eye, skin, and immune health. I particularly enjoy the vanilla-scented flavor of the fruit. Although there is no exact substitute, a crisp pear would be a lovely alternative out of season to counterbalance the bitterness of the endives. SERVES 4

FOR THE DRESSING

3 Tbsp (45 mL) extra virgin olive oil

1 Tbsp (15 mL) red wine vinegar

2 tsp (10 mL) honey

1 tsp (5 mL) Dijon mustard

1 shallot, minced

Salt and pepper

FOR THE SALAD

2 persimmons, peeled and thinly sliced

3 Belgian endives, halved and thickly sliced

3 Tbsp (45 mL) toasted and chopped pecans (see Nutrition Note)

2 Tbsp (30 mL) chopped fresh mint

1. **MAKE THE DRESSING** In a large bowl, whisk together the oil, vinegar, honey, mustard, and shallot. Season with salt and pepper.

2. **MAKE THE SALAD** Add the persimmons, endive, pecans, and mint and toss to mix. Serve immediately.

NUTRITION NOTE: Did you know that pecans contain more antioxidants than any other nut? Thanks to that, and to their healthy fat and high-fiber profile, they make for a wonderful snack or addition to your favorite recipes.

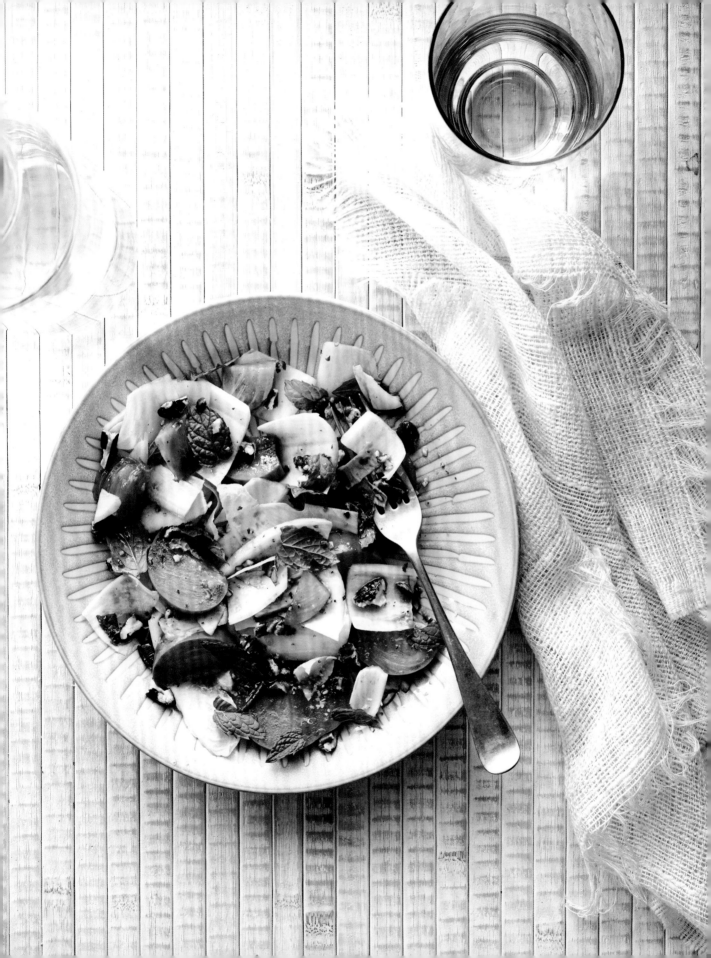

Kale Fattoush

Vegetarian • Dairy-free • Nut-free

With juicy vegetables, sweet pomegranate, crunchy pita, and fresh herbs, this salad is a real treat for the senses. Sturdy kale is the perfect addition to this classic salad, as it holds up well to the tangy and syrupy pomegranate molasses dressing. SERVES 6

FOR THE PITA CHIPS

3 medium whole wheat pitas

Olive oil

2 tsp (10 mL) za'atar, store-bought or homemade (page 245)

FOR THE SALAD

2 cups (500 mL) packed chopped kale

2 cups (500 mL) packed chopped romaine lettuce

1 cup (250 mL) finely chopped fresh flat-leaf parsley

1 cup (250 mL) finely chopped fresh mint

3 green onions, sliced

2 cups (500 mL) cherry tomatoes, halved

1 cup (250 mL) pomegranate arils (from 1 pomegranate)

4 radishes, sliced

3 Persian cucumbers, sliced

FOR THE DRESSING

Juice of ½ lemon

⅓ cup (80 mL) extra virgin olive oil

3 Tbsp (45 mL) pomegranate molasses

1 Tbsp (15 mL) honey

1 garlic clove, minced

2 tsp (10 mL) sumac

Salt and pepper

1. Preheat the oven to 400°F (200°C).

2. **MAKE THE PITA CHIPS** Brush the pitas with olive oil to coat, sprinkle with the za'atar, and place on a baking sheet. Bake for 8 to 10 minutes, until golden. Remove from the oven, let cool, and then break into small pieces. (See Kitchen Tip.)

3. **PREPARE THE SALAD** In a large bowl, gently toss together the kale, romaine, parsley, mint, green onions, tomatoes, pomegranate arils, radishes, and cucumber.

4. **MAKE THE DRESSING** In a liquid measuring cup, whisk together the lemon juice, oil, pomegranate molasses, honey, garlic, sumac, and salt and pepper to taste, until the dressing is emulsified.

5. Pour the dressing over the salad and toss, ensuring the kale is very well coated with the dressing. Allow the salad to rest 15 minutes, giving the kale time to tenderize. Garnish with the crispy pita chips and serve.

KITCHEN TIP: The pita chips can be made in advance. Store them in an airtight container at room temperature for up to 3 days.

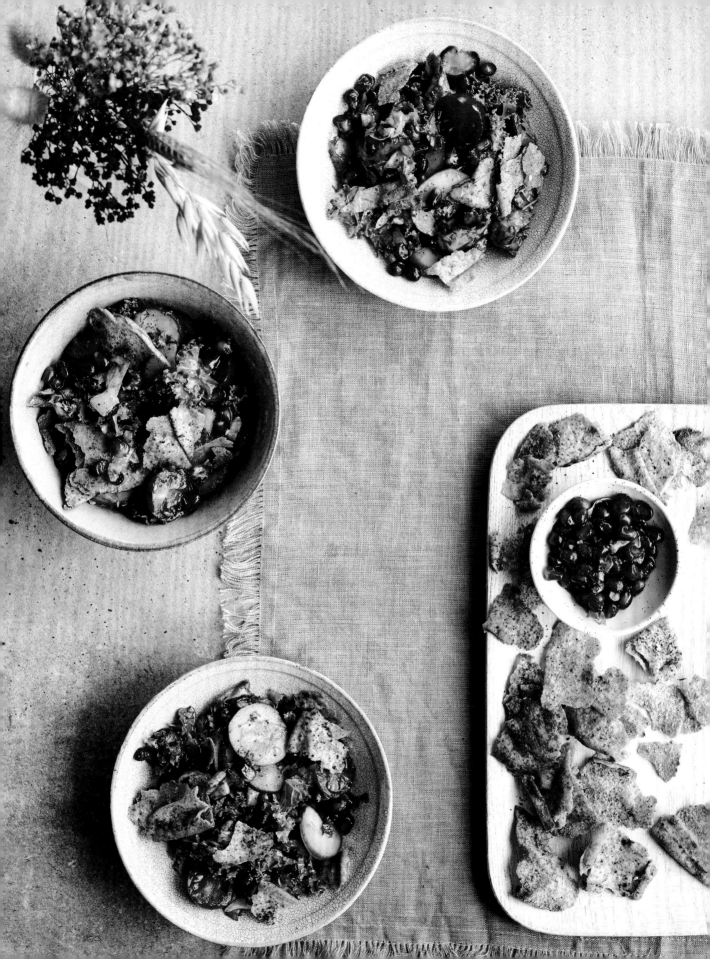

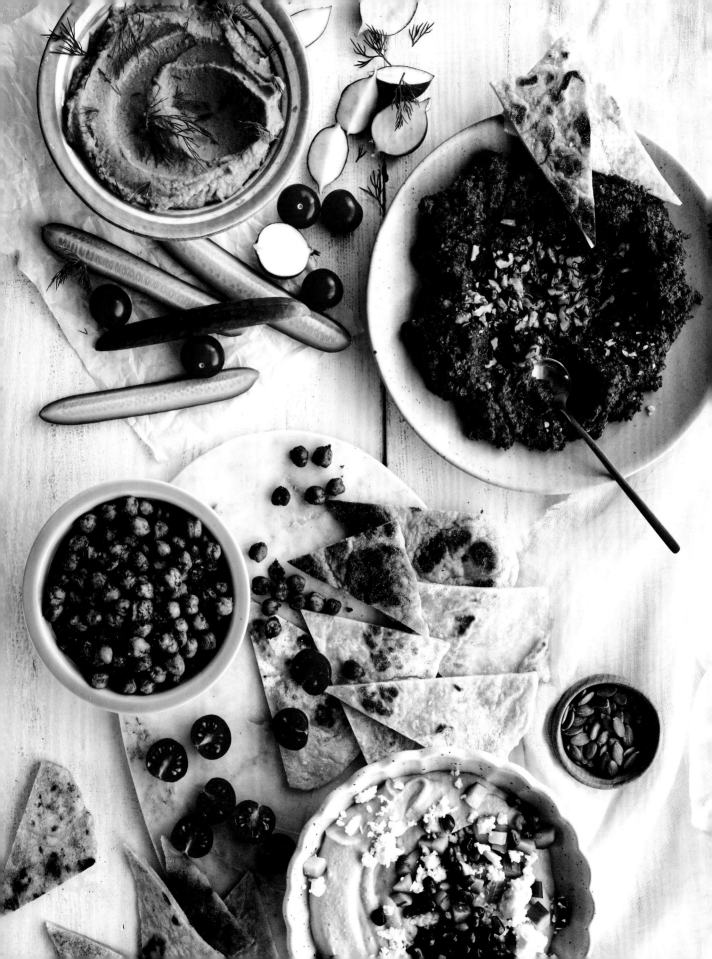

Bites and Appetizers

Every day is an excuse for an appetizer, in my book. And when they're this simple, you won't reserve them for special occasions. When I'm pressed for time, I like to make a meal of them—and take pleasure in watching guests relish the flavors from one bite to the next. Since these dishes are designed to be served before a main course, you can expect lots of vegetables, fresh herbs, and spices to feature in this chapter, in recipes that awaken your palate and appetite without overdoing it. You can also expect friends to quickly gather around the kitchen counter at the sight of these dishes, so be warned: these will go fast.

Dill and Avocado Hummus

Vegan • Vegetarian • Dairy-free • Gluten-free • Nut-free

Bright and zingy, the combination of lemon and dill makes this hummus-inspired dip come alive. I developed this recipe as an alternative for my son, who has a sesame allergy. In place of traditional tahini (sesame paste), avocado lends creaminess to this hummus, packing it with healthy fats and a beautiful green color, made even brighter by the fresh herbs. Serve this hummus with raw vegetables, or spread it on a slice of rye bread and garnish with smoked salmon for a flavorful hors-d'oeuvre. MAKES ABOUT 2 CUPS (500 ML)

1 can (19 oz/540 mL) chickpeas, drained but liquid reserved (see Kitchen Tip opposite)

1 garlic clove

1 ripe avocado, peeled and pitted

¼ cup (60 mL) fresh dill, plus more to garnish

Juice of 1 lemon

¼ cup (60 mL) chickpea liquid

Salt and pepper

Extra virgin olive oil, to serve

2 cucumbers, sliced into rounds, to serve

1 large pita, cut into wedges, to serve

1. Place the chickpeas in a large bowl, cover with water, and rub the chickpeas between your fingers to loosen the skin. As the skins float to the surface, tilt the bowl gently into the sink to discard them. Drain the chickpeas.

2. Place the chickpeas, garlic, avocado, dill, lemon juice, and chickpea liquid in a food processor fitted with a steel blade. Process until very smooth, 1 to 2 minutes. Season with salt and pepper.

3. Spread the hummus on a plate, drizzle with olive oil, and garnish with the dill. Serve with cucumber slices or pita wedges.

NUTRITION NOTE: Fresh herbs are prominent ingredients in the Mediterranean diet and add wonderful flavor to so many dishes. Interestingly, they are also quite rich in protective plant compounds, more than many fruit and vegetables! Don't shy away from them.

All-Dressed Hummus

Vegan · Vegetarian · Dairy-free · Gluten-free · Nut-free

This classic creamy dip gets an upgrade with the addition of crunchy cucumber, bursts of juicy pomegranate, and citrusy sumac. A feast for the eyes and the taste buds, colorful garnishes are perfect for a crowd. Feel free to add your own toppings keeping in mind textural variety (creamy, crunchy, juicy, etc.). Feta, tomato, pumpkin seeds, and/or za'atar would be lovely touches as well. MAKES ABOUT 2 CUPS (500 ML)

1. Place the chickpeas in a large bowl, cover with water, and rub the chickpeas between your fingers to loosen the skin. As the skins float to the surface, tilt the bowl gently into the sink to discard them. Drain the chickpeas.

2. Place the chickpeas, garlic, lemon juice, chickpea liquid, and tahini in a food processor fitted with a steel blade. Process until very smooth, 1 to 2 minutes. Season with salt and pepper.

3. Spread the hummus on a serving plate and drizzle with the oil. Top with the pomegranate arils, cucumber, and a generous dusting of sumac.

KITCHEN TIP: Save that liquid! The liquid from the chickpea can, also known as aquafaba, helps give the hummus a creamy consistency.

1 can (19 oz/540 mL) chickpeas, drained but liquid reserved (see Kitchen Tip)

2 garlic cloves

Juice of 1 lemon

¼ cup (60 mL) chickpea liquid

¼ cup (60 mL) tahini

Salt and pepper

Extra virgin olive oil

¼ cup (60 mL) pomegranate arils

2 Persian cucumbers, finely diced

¼ to ½ tsp (1 to 2.5 mL) sumac

Muhammara

Vegan • Vegetarian • Dairy-free

The first time I tasted muhammara, I could hardly believe my taste buds. The combination of peppers, walnuts, warming spices, and pomegranate molasses (a uniquely tangy syrup made from concentrated pomegranate juice) is what makes you keep coming back for more. Nutritionally, this spread is a wonderful way to include more walnuts—a source of plant-based omega-3 fats—in your diet. Also, because its flavor is so complex, it is the ideal dip to encourage vegetable intake. For the sake of time, I use store-bought roasted peppers for this recipe and also tomato paste, as it is more flavorful than most tomatoes we have access to year-round. MAKES ABOUT 1¼ CUPS (310 ML)

½ cup (125 mL) raw walnuts

¼ cup (60 mL) plain breadcrumbs, store-bought (such as panko) or homemade (page 244)

1 cup (250 mL) store-bought jarred roasted red peppers

2 Tbsp (30 mL) tomato paste

1 Tbsp (15 mL) Aleppo pepper (see Kitchen Tip)

1 tsp (5 mL) paprika

½ tsp (2.5 mL) ground cumin

1 garlic clove, minced

1 Tbsp (15 mL) pomegranate molasses

1 Tbsp (15 mL) tahini

2 Tbsp (30 mL) extra virgin olive oil, plus more to serve

Salt

Flatbreads (page 109) (optional)

1. In a small, dry skillet set over medium heat, toast the nuts until fragrant, tossing frequently, about 5 minutes. Transfer the nuts to a cutting board and let cool slightly. Finely chop and set aside in a large bowl.

2. In the same pan, add the breadcrumbs and toast until golden, 2–3 minutes. Transfer to the bowl containing the nuts.

3. In a food processor fitted with a steel blade, process the roasted peppers, tomato paste, Aleppo pepper, paprika, cumin, garlic, pomegranate molasses, and tahini for 1 minute or until smooth. Using a spatula, scrape all the pepper mixture from the bowl of the processor and add it to the nut mixture. Stir to combine. The consistency will be thick but spreadable.

4. Add the oil and stir to combine. Season with salt. Spread the muhammara on a serving plate, drizzle with more olive oil, and serve with fresh flatbreads.

KITCHEN TIP: Aleppo pepper is fragrant, not spicy, and slightly sweet. It's increasingly available in grocery stores, and is easily found online.

Greek Yogurt Flatbreads

Vegetarian • Nut-free

Tender and flavorful, these simple flatbreads require no kneading or resting. They make the perfect accompaniment to your favorite classic Mediterranean dishes, like the Pork Souvlaki Pitas (page 192), or the hummus dips (pages 106 and 107). You can also use these flatbreads as a quick pizza base, topped with seasonal vegetables, or keep it simple and serve with a plate of olive oil sprinkled with za'atar. They are delicious, versatile, and can be made in advance, should you be pressed for time. MAKES 8 FLATBREADS

1. Place the yogurt, oil, and salt in a large bowl and stir to combine. Stir in the flour and baking powder, mixing well.

2. Flour a work surface and a rolling pin. Turn the dough onto the work surface and shape it with your hands to form a ball. Divide into eight equal pieces, and roll out each piece into a 6-inch (15 cm) disc.

3. Heat a large 12-inch (30 cm) non-stick skillet over high heat. Add the discs, one at a time, and cook until bubbly and browned, 1 to 2 minutes per side. Serve. Store the flatbreads in a resealable bag at room temperature for 1 to 2 days, or in the freezer for up to 2 months. To reheat, defrost the pitas and warm them in a dry pan before serving.

2 cups (500 mL) plain Greek yogurt

¼ cup (60 mL) extra virgin olive oil

½ tsp (2.5 mL) kosher salt

2½ cups (625 mL) spelt or all-purpose flour

1 tsp (5 mL) baking powder

Spiced Roasted Chickpeas

Vegan • Vegetarian • Dairy-free • Gluten-free • Nut-free

These crispy chickpeas are wonderful for nibbling with guests over cocktails, but I particularly enjoy them as a midday snack. They satisfy a crunch craving and, given their protein and fiber content, are filling too. Seasoned with ras el hanout, a fragrant and warming Moroccan spice mixture, these chickpeas pack a lot of flavor. You can also add them as a textural component in dishes like soups and salads for extra crunch.

MAKES ABOUT 2 CUPS (500 ML)

1 can (19 oz/540 mL) chickpeas, drained and rinsed

1 Tbsp (15 mL) olive oil

2 tsp (10 mL) ras el hanout (see Kitchen Tip)

Salt and pepper

1. Preheat the oven to 375°F (190°C) (use convection setting or for further advice, see page 61). Line a baking sheet with parchment paper.

2. Place the chickpeas in a large bowl, cover with water, and rub the chickpeas between your fingers to loosen the skin. As the skins float to the surface, tilt the bowl gently into the sink to discard the skins. Drain the chickpeas, lay them on a clean kitchen towel, and pat them as dry as possible with another clean kitchen towel. Then allow them to air-dry for 15 minutes.

3. In a bowl, combine the chickpeas, oil, and ras el hanout. Season with salt and pepper. Toss and spread evenly on the prepared baking sheet.

4. Bake for 45 to 50 minutes, stirring every 15 minutes, until the chickpeas are crispy and golden. Allow the chickpeas to cool completely before storing them; they will continue to crisp up as they cool. Any leftovers can be stored in an airtight container at room temperature for up to 1 week.

KITCHEN TIP: You can find ras el hanout in the spice section of your local grocery store or quite easily online.

Sweet and Savory Roasted Nuts with Rosemary and Honey

Vegetarian • Dairy-free • Gluten-free

These addictive nuts are fragrant, spicy, and sweet. I like to make a batch when I entertain to zhuzh up a cheeseboard, and I'll snack on the leftovers during the week (that is, if there *are* any leftovers). Nuts are prominent in Mediterranean cuisine and contribute heart-healthy fats to your diet. Aim to eat a handful a few times per week—the amount shown to have a positive impact on health. Keeping with the Mediterranean spirit of hospitality, you can wrap any extra nuts as take-home gifts for guests, a greatly appreciated gesture, as they're often devoured on the way home! MAKES 4 CUPS (1 L)

1. Preheat the oven to 325°F (165°C). Line a large baking sheet with parchment paper.

2. In a large bowl, toss the walnuts, cashews, and almonds with the rosemary, cayenne pepper, and salt to taste.

3. Place the oil and honey in a liquid measuring cup. Warm in the microwave for 30 seconds, then whisk to combine. Pour over the nuts and toss to coat.

4. Spread the nuts evenly on the prepared baking sheet. Bake for 12 to 15 minutes, stirring halfway through, until the nuts are golden brown. Adjust the seasoning to taste, and let cool completely before serving. Any leftovers can be stored in an airtight container at room temperature for up to 1 week or in the freezer for up to 1 month.

2 cups (500 mL) raw walnuts

1 cup (250 mL) raw cashews

1 cup (250 mL) raw almonds

3 Tbsp (45 mL) minced rosemary

½ tsp (2.5 mL) cayenne pepper

Salt

2 Tbsp (30 mL) olive oil

2 Tbsp (30 mL) honey

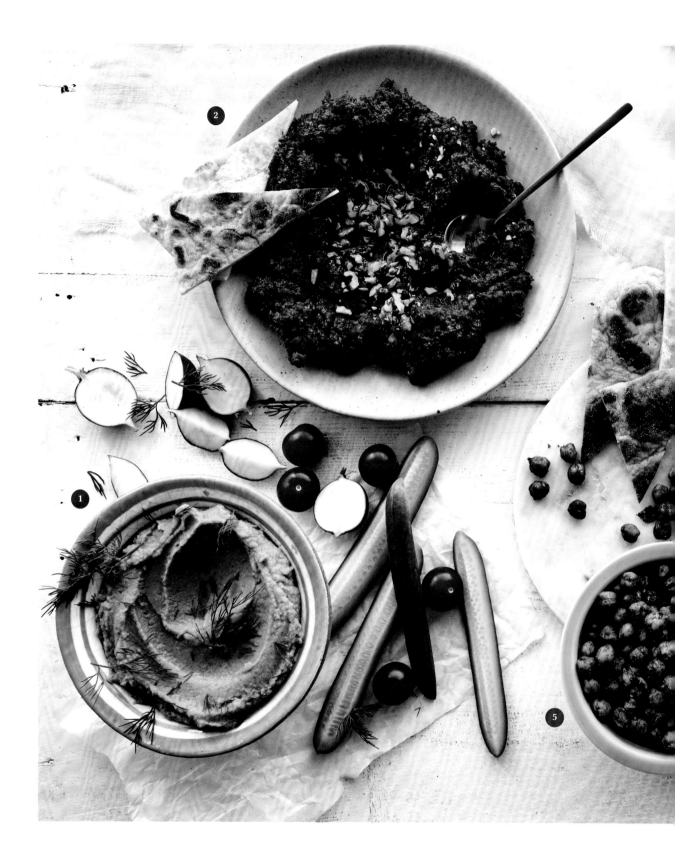

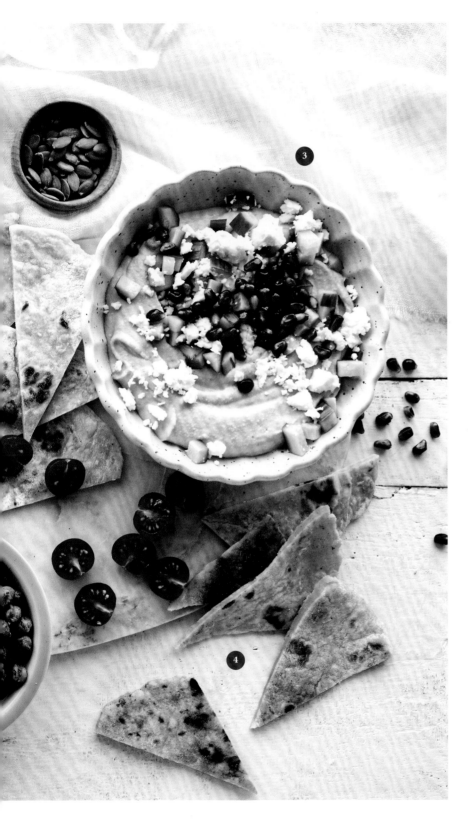

Marinated Carrots with Mint and Honey

Vegetarian • Dairy-free • Gluten-free • Nut-free

The combination of sweet and tangy pickled carrots with the fresh mint and floral honey is highly addictive. I like to serve these palate-awakening carrots with an antipasto course.
SERVES 8 TO 10

6 cups (1.5 L) water

3 cups (750 mL) white vinegar

Salt

2 lb (1 kg) Nantes or other small to medium carrots, peeled and halved lengthwise

3 to 4 Tbsp (45 to 60 mL) extra virgin olive oil

2 Tbsp (30 mL) honey

Pepper

2 Tbsp (30 mL) chopped fresh mint

1. In a large pot, combine the water, vinegar, and a generous pinch of salt. Bring to a boil, reduce to a simmer, and add the carrots. Cook for 15 minutes or until the carrots are tender but still have a bite. Drain and transfer to a bowl.

2. While they're still hot, toss the carrots in the oil (enough to coat them well) and honey. Season with salt and pepper. Let cool to room temperature.

3. Add the mint, toss, and serve. Any leftovers can be stored in an airtight jar or container in the refrigerator for up to 1 week.

Olives with Fennel and Chili

Vegan • Vegetarian • Dairy-free • Gluten-free • Nut-free

These black, wrinkly olives pack big flavor. They also come with all the benefits that olive oil is known for. They make a fine snack on their own, but are also delicious added to the Fennel and Orange Salad (page 96) and to pasta dishes, or mixed with fresh tomatoes to accompany grilled fish. MAKES 2 CUPS (500 ML)

2 cups (500 mL) sun-dried black olives

1 tsp (5 mL) fennel seeds

¼ cup (60 mL) extra virgin olive oil

¼ tsp (1 mL) crushed chili flakes

1. Place the olives in a bowl and cover with water. Let soak for 1 hour. Drain and repeat this step until the olives no longer taste excessively salty. This may take two or four rinses, depending on how salty they were to start. Drain the olives and pat them with paper towel until completely dry.

2. In a small, dry skillet set over medium heat, toast the fennel seeds until fragrant, about 2 minutes.

3. In a large bowl, toss the olives with the oil, fennel seeds, and chili flakes. Any leftovers can be stored in an airtight jar or container in the refrigerator for up to 1 month.

Marinated Mushrooms with Chili and Parsley

Vegan · Vegetarian · Dairy-free · Gluten-free · Nut-free

If you are a mushroom lover, this recipe is for you. I'm a fan myself, as nothing quite beats their earthy flavor and versatility in the kitchen. Your taste buds will fall in love all over again with this scrumptious vegetable, thanks to the surprising hit of acid and heat. These are easy to make and always a hit at gatherings. MAKES 4 CUPS (1 L)

1. In a large saucepan, bring the water, vinegar, and a generous pinch of salt to a boil. Reduce the heat to medium, and add the mushrooms. Cook for 10 minutes or until a sharp knife can easily pierce the stems. Drain and shake off any excess water.

2. While they're still hot, toss the mushrooms in the oil (enough to coat them) and chili flakes, stirring well to coat. Season with salt and pepper, and let cool. Stir in the parsley and serve. Any leftovers can be stored in an airtight jar or container in the refrigerator for up to 1 month.

6 cups (1.5 L) water

3 cups (750 mL) white vinegar

Salt

2 packages (8 oz/227 g each) miniature or small button mushrooms, quartered

3 to 4 Tbsp (45 to 60 mL) extra virgin olive oil

¼ tsp (1 mL) crushed chili flakes

Pepper

2 Tbsp (30 mL) chopped fresh flat-leaf parsley

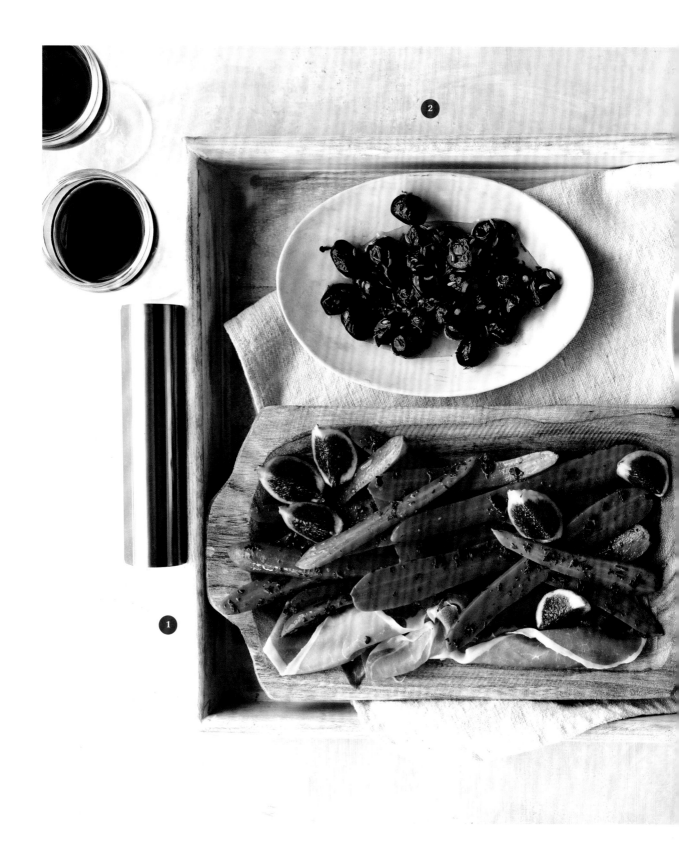

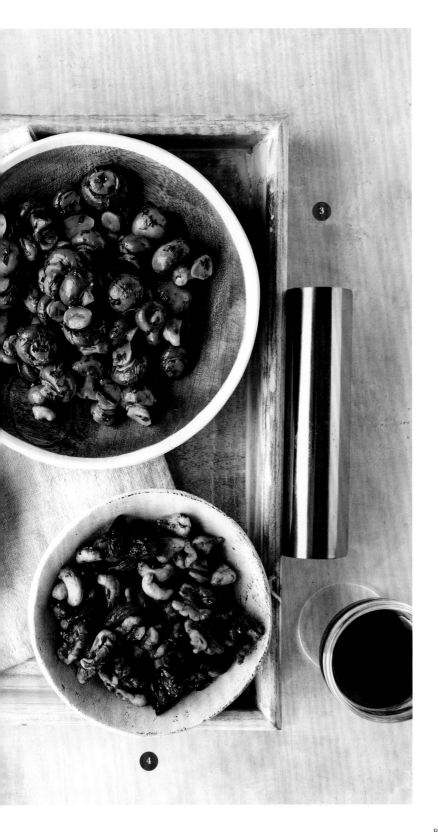

1. Marinated Carrots with Mint and Honey (page 114)

2. Olives with Fennel and Chili (page 114)

3. Marinated Mushrooms with Chili and Parsley (page 115)

4. Sweet and Savory Roasted Nuts with Rosemary and Honey (page 111)

Delicata Squash Rings with Labneh Dip

Vegetarian • Gluten-free • Nut-free

Faithful to the Mediterranean practice of eating in season, I am always on the hunt for creative ways to make use of the abundant squash we have in the fall. Delicata squash has a lovely sweet flavor and is also practical—the skin is completely edible, so you can skip the peeling. In this dish, the squash is paired with fragrant herbs and spices, such as dried rosemary, cayenne, and chives, mainstays in Mediterranean cuisine for their flavor-enhancing abilities. Herbs and spices also display impressive antioxidant potential, and every sprinkle counts. The sweet-and-spicy squash rings, paired with the creamy and savory dip, make for a memorable dish that will be quickly devoured. SERVES 6

FOR THE SQUASH

2 small delicata squash, washed

2 Tbsp (30 mL) olive oil

2 Tbsp (30 mL) cornstarch

2 Tbsp (30 mL) dried rosemary

¼ tsp (1 mL) cayenne pepper

Salt and pepper

FOR THE DIP

1 cup (250 mL) labneh

3 Tbsp (45 mL) finely chopped chives

1 garlic clove, minced

2 Tbsp (30 mL) extra virgin olive oil

Juice of ½ lemon

Salt and pepper

1. Preheat the oven to 400°F (200°C). Place two baking sheets in the oven to heat.

2. **MAKE THE SQUASH** Trim the ends off the squash and spoon out the seeds, forming a hollowed cylinder. Thinly slice the squash using a mandoline (set at ⅛ inch/3 mm) (see Kitchen Tip).

3. In a large bowl, toss the sliced squash with the oil, cornstarch, rosemary, cayenne pepper, and salt and pepper to taste.

4. Carefully remove the hot baking sheets from the oven and spread the squash on each in an even layer. Bake for 15 minutes, flipping the squash halfway through and rotating the baking sheets. When browned, remove from the oven and let cool on the baking sheet.

5. **MAKE THE DIP** In a small bowl, combine the labneh, chives, garlic, oil, and lemon juice. Season with salt and pepper.

6. Serve the squash rings with the dip. Leftover squash and dip can be stored in individual airtight containers in the refrigerator for up to 3 days.

KITCHEN TIP: The mandoline is ideal for creating even slices. However, a sharp knife will also do the trick.

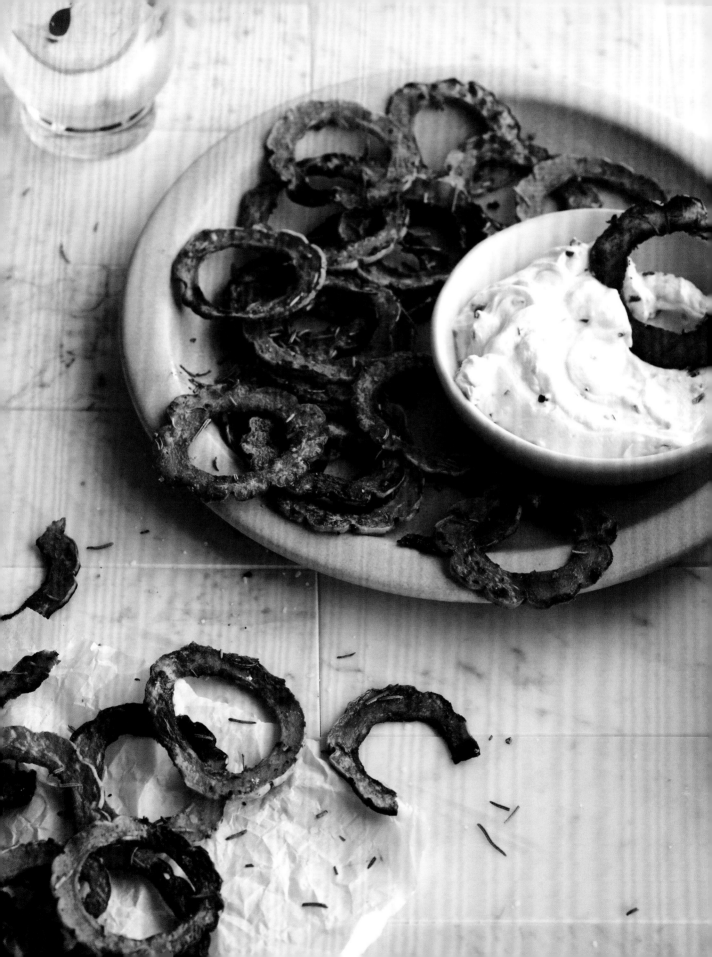

Escarole and White Bean Toasts

Vegan • Vegetarian • Dairy-free • Nut-free

The bitterness of escarole is mellowed out in the cooking process, developing an almost silky texture and sweet flavor. Paired with lemon, garlic, chili, and creamy beans, these little toasts, or crostini, make a delightful winter appetizer. Although this recipe lends itself well to feeding a crowd, its bolstering fiber and protein, thanks to the formidable duo of beans and greens, means it can just as easily serve as a balanced, plant-based meal. For a party of one, simply swap the baguette for a larger slice of crusty sourdough. SERVES 4

3 Tbsp (45 mL) olive oil, divided

1 head escarole, chopped

4 garlic cloves, sliced

1 red Italian Long Hot pepper, seeded and sliced

Peel of ½ lemon, julienned

1 can (19 oz/540 mL) cannellini beans, drained and rinsed

¾ cup (180 mL) water

Salt and pepper

1 baguette, sliced into ½-inch-thick (1.2 cm) slices

1. Heat 1 Tbsp (15 mL) oil in a 12-inch (30 cm) non-stick skillet set over medium-high heat. Add the escarole and cook for 5 minutes, stirring until it wilts. Transfer to a plate.

2. In the same skillet set over medium, heat the remaining 2 Tbsp (30 mL) oil. Add the garlic, hot pepper, and lemon peel and cook for 1 minute or until fragrant. Add the beans and water. Cook for 5 minutes or until it's a creamy consistency and most of the moisture has absorbed.

3. Return the escarole to the skillet, season with salt and pepper, and cook for 5 minutes more. Meanwhile, toast the bread.

4. Spread the bean and escarole mixture on the toasted bread, and serve. Any leftovers can be stored in an airtight container in the refrigerator for up to 3 days.

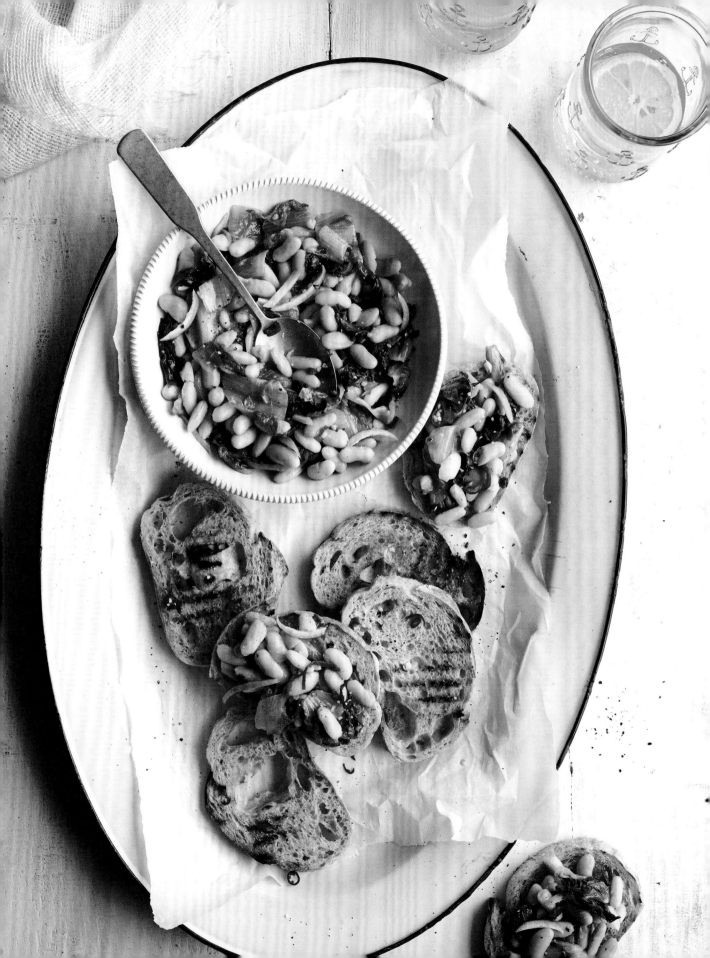

Rainbow Wraps with Swiss Chard and Halloumi

Vegetarian • Gluten-free • Nut-free

Swiss chard is a beloved Mediterranean green and, notably, an excellent source of vitamins A and K. I remember my grandfather harvesting and filling entire bags of Swiss chard for my family every week as he kept up with his garden. As a new gardener, I've found Swiss chard to be one of my most successful crops, which is why I'm always thinking up ways to prepare it. In this dish, a quick blanch turns the chard leaves into pliable, buttery wraps. These bundles are filled to the brim with crunchy vegetables—including tangy marinated turnips—salty olives, and halloumi. Your go-to app for your next get-together or favorite new vegetarian lunch option! MAKES 4 WRAPS

4 large Swiss chard leaves

3 oz (85 g) halloumi, cut into 8 slices

½ cup (125 mL) fresh mint

½ cup (125 mL) green olives, pitted and sliced

½ cup (125 mL) store-bought pickled turnips

1 carrot, peeled and cut into thin 3-inch-long (8 cm) strips

1 red bell pepper, cut into thin 3-inch-long (8 cm) strips

1 English cucumber, cut into thin 3-inch-long (8 cm) strips

Tahini sauce, store-bought or homemade (page 249)

1. Bring a large pot of water to a boil. Blanch the chard leaves for 1 minute, then shock them in ice water and transfer to a work surface.

2. In a grill pan set over high heat, grill the halloumi until grill marks appear, about 1 to 2 minutes per side.

3. Trim the stem of the chard. Place two slices of cheese in the center of a chard leaf and top with a layer of mint, olives, turnip, and three to four strips each of carrot, pepper, and cucumber, being mindful not to overstuff so the wraps remain easy to roll. Fold the outer sides of the chard toward the center and roll firmly, tucking in the filings. Repeat with the remaining leaves and the remainder of the fillings. Cut in half widthwise and serve with the tahini sauce.

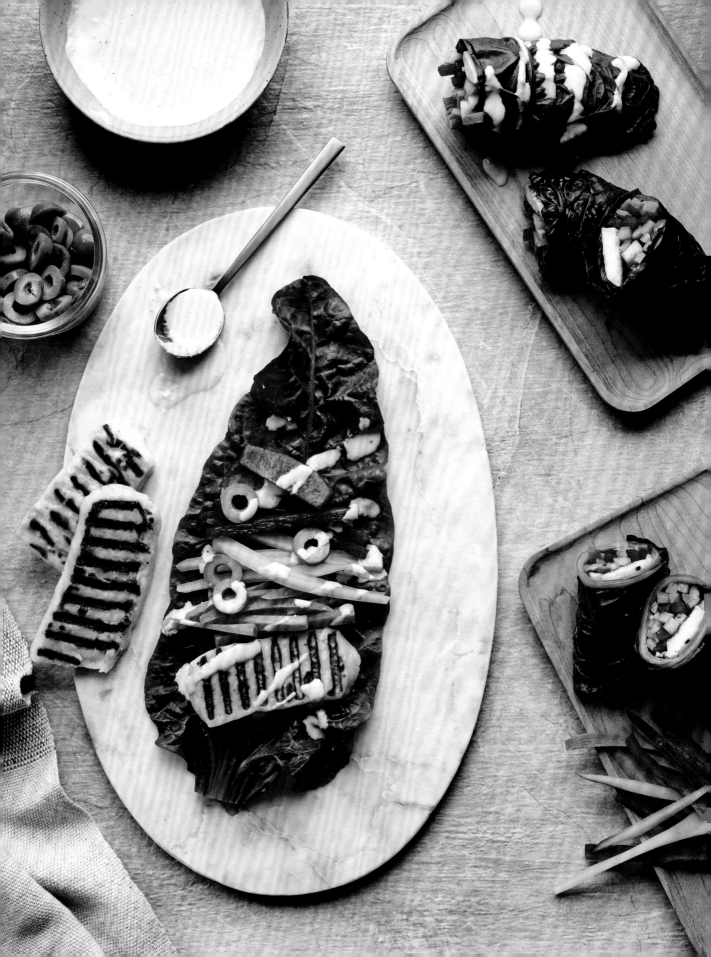

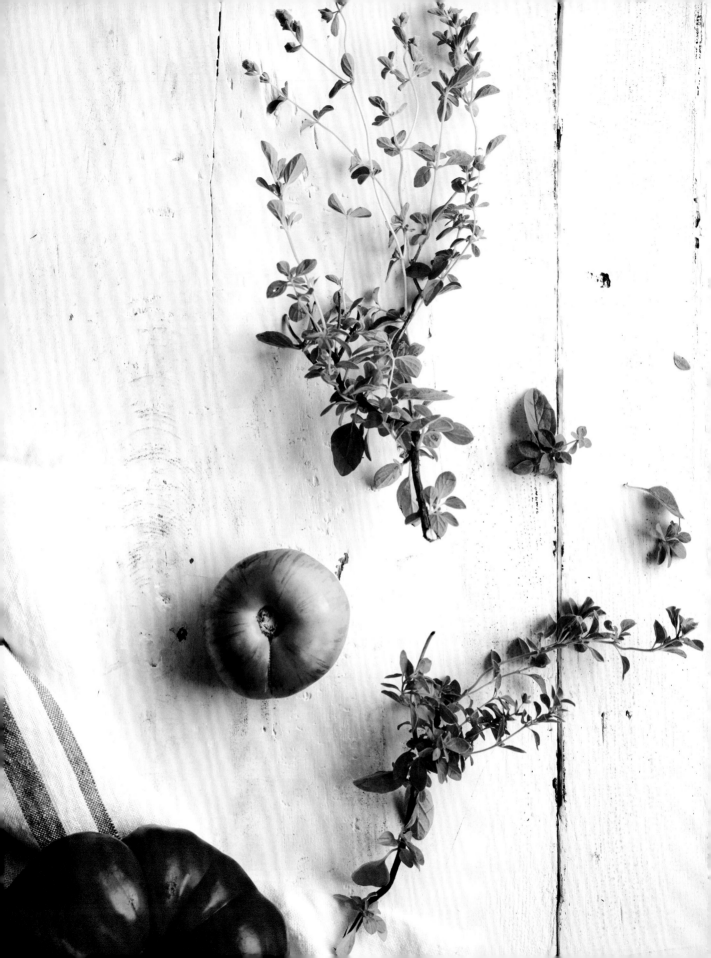

Sides

Side dishes shine as bright as mains in Mediterranean cuisine, as they often showcase beautiful, seasonal vegetables. As discussed in Principle 6, enjoy plant-centric meals (page 28), vegetables have a lot to offer in terms of nutrition, notably in the form of gut-friendly fiber and disease-protecting phytonutrients. In this chapter, colorful and mouth-watering vegetable-based dishes take the stage, to inspire you to live out this principle at every meal, and to love every bite.

Couscous with Shallots, Pistachios, and Currants

Vegan • Vegetarian • Dairy-free

Couscous is an everyday pantry staple I quite enjoy. It cooks quickly and takes on whatever flavor you throw at it. But contrary to what you may think, couscous is *not* a whole grain. Rather, it's a type of pasta, meaning it doesn't bolster meals with the same high fiber content as some of its whole grain counterparts. Whole wheat couscous has the nutritional edge, so choose that if you can find it. But if you can't, know that plain couscous still works well, especially when paired with filling high-fiber ingredients like the ones in this recipe. Savory shallots, crunchy pistachios, sweet currants, and fresh mint turn plain couscous into a delicious speedy side. SERVES 4

1 cup (250 mL) couscous (preferably whole wheat)

Salt

2 Tbsp (30 mL) olive oil

6 shallots, sliced (about 1½ cups/375 mL)

¼ cup (60 mL) chopped fresh mint

¼ cup (60 mL) unsalted pistachios, toasted

3 Tbsp (45 mL) currants or raisins

Juice of ½ lemon

1. Place the couscous in a large bowl. Bring 1 cup (250 mL) water to a boil and pour over the couscous. Add a pinch of salt, stir, cover, and let sit for 5 to 10 minutes for the water to absorb.

2. Heat the oil in a 10-inch (25 cm) non-stick skillet set over medium-low heat. Add the shallots and cook until caramelized, about 15 minutes, stirring often and adding 1 to 2 Tbsp (15 to 30 mL) water if the shallots dry up, to prevent burning.

3. Add the shallots and their cooking oil to the couscous, then the mint, pistachios, currants, and lemon juice. Gently toss and serve. Any leftovers can be stored in an airtight container in the refrigerator for up to 3 days.

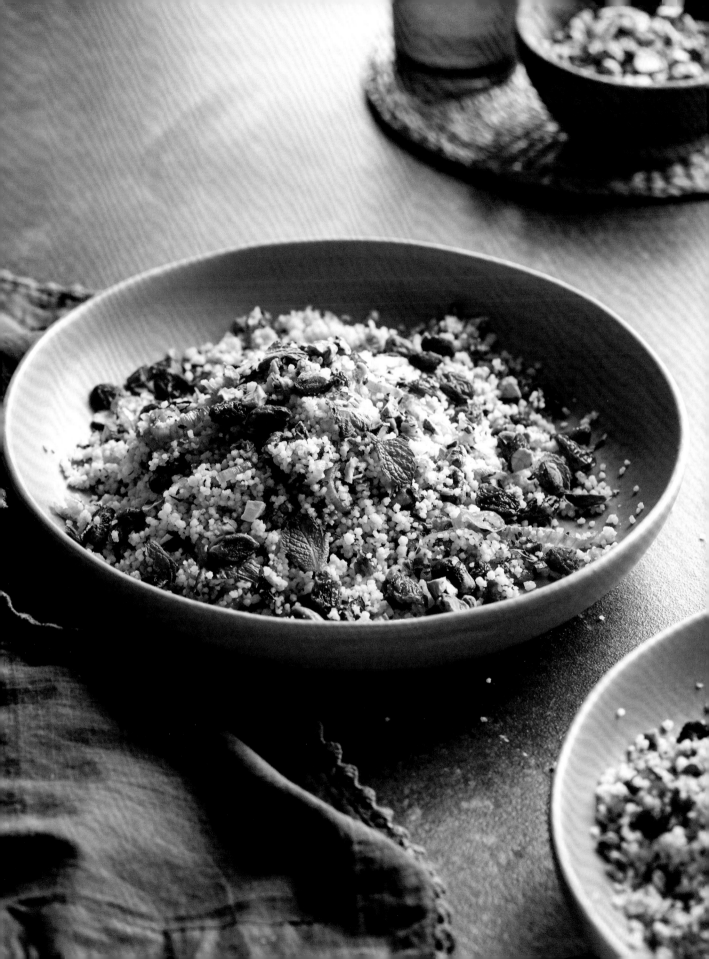

Eggplant Wedges with Roasted Garlic Vinaigrette

Vegetarian • Dairy-free • Gluten-free • Nut-free

The transformation that garlic undergoes when it's roasted—from sharp to mellow yet complex, with a buttery texture to boot—has always amazed me. It's worth the wait. In this recipe, once the roasted garlic comes out of the oven, you will squeeze the caramelized flesh into a blender and blitz it into a zippy olive oil and lemon dressing. It's perfect for drizzling over the roasted eggplant wedges. I love to serve these as a part of an antipasto platter or alongside pasta, including my Bolognese with Lentils and Mushrooms (page 162). SERVES 4 TO 6

FOR THE VINAIGRETTE

1 garlic bulb

1 tsp (5 mL) plus ⅓ cup (80 mL) extra virgin olive oil, divided

Salt and pepper

Juice of 1 lemon

1 tsp (5 mL) honey

FOR THE EGGPLANT

2 eggplant (about 1 lb/450 g each), cut into wedges (see Kitchen Tip)

3 Tbsp (45 mL) olive oil

Salt and pepper

10 basil leaves, coarsely chopped

1 red Italian Long Hot pepper, seeded and sliced

1. Preheat the oven to 375°F (190°C). Line a baking sheet with parchment paper.

2. **MAKE THE VINAIGRETTE** Slice off the top of the garlic bulb to expose the cloves. Drizzle with 1 tsp (5 mL) olive oil, add a pinch of salt and pepper, and wrap tightly in aluminum foil. Bake for 45 minutes. Let cool before handling.

3. Increase the oven temperature to 400°F (200°C).

4. **MAKE THE EGGPLANT** Brush the eggplant with the oil and season with salt and pepper. Place the wedges, skin side down, on the prepared baking sheet. Bake for 20 to 25 minutes, until golden brown.

5. To make the vinaigrette, squeeze the roasted garlic out of the skins and into a blender. Add the lemon juice and honey, start the motor on the lowest setting, and slowly pour in the remaining ⅓ cup (80 mL) oil, continuing to blend and increasing the speed until the vinaigrette is emulsified. Season with salt and pepper, and pulse one more time to combine.

6. Arrange the eggplant wedges on a plate, drizzle with vinaigrette, then garnish with the basil and hot pepper. Any leftover vinaigrette can be stored in an airtight container in the refrigerator for up to 3 days. Leftover eggplant can be stored in an airtight container in the refrigerator for up to 2 days.

KITCHEN TIP: A trick I learned from my grandmother too late in life: store eggplant at room temperature, stem side down, in a container filled with about ½ inch (1.2 cm) water. They will stay fresh for up to 5 days.

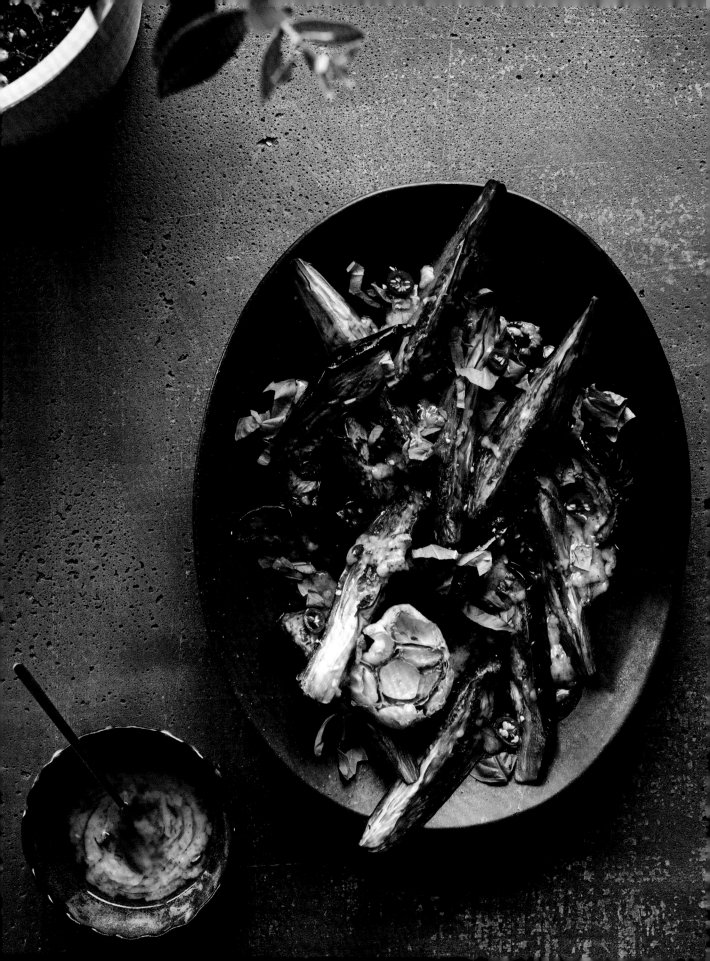

Swiss Chard with Crispy Breadcrumbs

Vegetarian • Nut-free

One of the most impactful routines I learned growing up was that of vegetable prep. On the weekend, my family would blanch their abundant vegetables and store them in the refrigerator. Containers of Swiss chard, kale, and rapini filled the shelves. Then, during the week, all that needed to be done was quickly sauté the vegetables in olive oil. This made it easy to ensure that a pile of greens was present with every single meal. This recipe is inspired by that practice. The Swiss chard is cooked, then sautéed and topped with crispy breadcrumbs. The first step can be done in advance and you can enjoy this side in minutes, even on weekdays. SERVES 4

2 bunches of Swiss chard leaves, chopped

2 Tbsp (30 mL) olive oil, divided

⅓ cup (80 mL) breadcrumbs, store-bought (such as panko) or homemade (page 244)

½ tsp (2.5 mL) crushed chili flakes

4 garlic cloves, sliced

3 Tbsp (45 mL) grated Pecorino Romano

1. Bring a large pot of water to a boil. Blanch the chard leaves for 2 minutes, then shock them in ice water to halt the cooking. Drain and reserve.

2. Heat 1 Tbsp (15 mL) oil in a 12-inch (30 cm) non-stick skillet set over medium heat. Add the breadcrumbs and chili flakes and toast for 1 to 2 minutes, until golden brown. Transfer to a bowl.

3. In the same pan set over medium, heat the remaining 1 Tbsp (15 mL) oil. Add the garlic and sauté until fragrant, 1 minute. Add the Swiss chard and sauté for 5 minutes or until the chard has warmed and is coated with the oil. Add the Pecorino, toss, and remove from the heat.

4. Sprinkle the chard with the breadcrumbs and serve. Store the chard in an airtight container in the refrigerator for up to 3 days. Store the breadcrumbs in an airtight container at room temperature for up to 3 days.

Grilled Vegetables

Vegan • Vegetarian • Dairy-free • Gluten-free • Nut-free

The versatility of grilled vegetables is unmatched. They can accompany your weeknight main, be served as part of an antipasto platter, jazz up a plain sandwich, or turn your next salad into something memorable. They also happen to be a wonderful make-ahead option, meaning you can prepare this recipe during your Sunday meal-prep routine and enjoy it throughout the week in various ways. Don't let the season hold you back; this recipe can also be made using a grill pan indoors, working in batches, for year-round grilled vegetables. SERVES 10

1. Preheat the barbecue or grill pan to medium-high and oil the grates.

2. Place the vegetables on a tray and brush with olive oil on all sides. Season with salt and pepper.

3. Transfer to the grill, laying them across the grates. Grill with the lid closed for 7 to 10 minutes, turning halfway through once grill marks appear and the vegetables begin to soften.

4. Place the vegetables on a large serving platter and drizzle with the vinaigrette. Garnish with the oregano and serve. Any leftover vegetables can be stored in an airtight container in the refrigerator for up to 4 days. The vinaigrette can be stored in the refrigerator for up to 1 week.

3 zucchini, sliced lengthwise into ½-inch-thick (1.2 cm) slices

1 eggplant, sliced lengthwise into ½-inch-thick (1.2 cm) slices

1 package (8 oz/227 g) cremini mushrooms

2 red onions, sliced into ½-inch-thick (1.2 cm) rings

1 bunch of asparagus, ends trimmed

2 red bell peppers, cored and quartered

2 orange bell peppers, cored and quartered

Olive oil

Salt and pepper

Balsamic Vinaigrette (page 246)

3 Tbsp (45 mL) fresh oregano

Braised Flat Beans with Tomatoes and Basil

Vegan • Vegetarian • Dairy-free • Gluten-free • Nut-free

As a child, I was fascinated by the climbing bean plants that overran my grandfather's fence. Romano beans are broad and flat, and typically longer than string beans. They are crunchy when raw and, when cooked, they have a meaty texture that soaks up flavor. In this dish, hearty romano beans are stewed in a jammy tomato and basil-kissed sauce. This makes a wonderful summer side dish to accompany simple grilled proteins, or you can toss these saucy beans with spaghetti for a memorable pasta dish. Since flat bean season is so short-lived, I tend to use green beans during the year, a substitute that works beautifully in this recipe. SERVES 4 TO 6

2 Tbsp (30 mL) olive oil

2 cups (500 mL) thinly sliced onion

3 garlic cloves, sliced

1 red Italian Long Hot pepper, seeded and sliced

1 lb (450 g) romano or green beans, trimmed

1 can (14 oz/398 mL) diced tomatoes

1 cup (250 mL) packed fresh basil

½ cup (125 mL) water

Salt and pepper

1. Heat the oil in a 12-inch (30 cm) non-stick skillet set over medium heat. Add the onion and soften for 7 minutes. Add the garlic and hot pepper, and cook for 1 minute or until fragrant. Stir in the beans and cook for 2 minutes.

2. Add the tomatoes, basil, water, and salt and pepper to taste. Toss to mix, cover, and reduce the heat to medium-low. Simmer for 20 to 25 minutes, stirring occasionally, until the beans are tender. Adjust the seasoning and serve. Any leftovers can be stored in an airtight container in the refrigerator for up to 3 days.

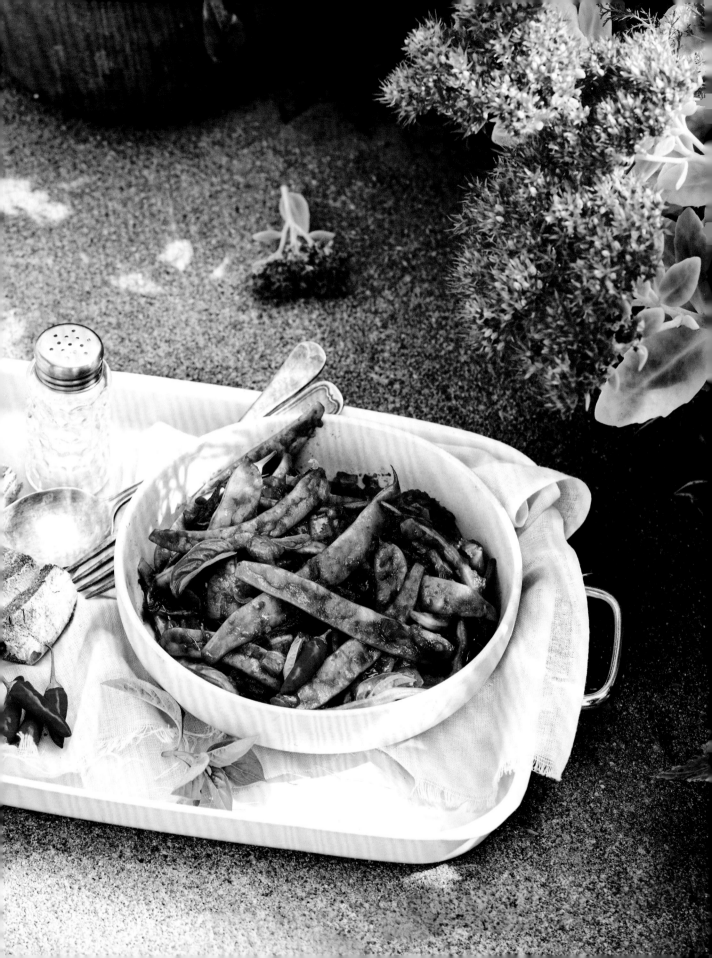

Bulgur and Roasted Brussels Sprouts, Tangerine, and Pomegranate

Vegetarian • Dairy-free • Nut-free

Bulgur is a whole grain in the wheat family that can easily replace rice or quinoa if you're looking to switch things up. It has a chewy, nutty texture and a flavor that lets other ingredients shine. In this dish, Brussels sprouts add even more gut-friendly fiber and a smoky flavor that works wonderfully. Serve with fish, such as my Baked Salmon with Gremolata Crust (page 182). SERVES 4 TO 6

FOR THE SALAD

1 lb (450 g) Brussels sprouts, trimmed

1 Tbsp (15 mL) olive oil

Salt and pepper

1 cup (250 mL) bulgur

1¾ cups (430 mL) water

½ cup (125 mL) pomegranate arils

1 tangerine, peeled and sliced into rounds

1 green onion, sliced

¼ cup (60 mL) finely chopped fresh mint

FOR THE DRESSING

2 Tbsp (30 mL) extra virgin olive oil

2 Tbsp (30 mL) white wine vinegar

1 tsp (5 mL) Dijon mustard

1 tsp (5 mL) honey

Salt and pepper

1. Preheat the oven to 425°F (220°C). Line a baking sheet with parchment paper.

2. MAKE THE SALAD In a food processor fitted with a steel blade, shred the Brussels sprouts. Transfer to the prepared baking sheet. Drizzle with the oil, season with salt and pepper, and toss to coat. Spread evenly on the baking sheet and bake for 12 to 15 minutes, until caramelized.

3. In a saucepan, bring the bulgur, water, and a pinch of salt to a boil, reduce to a simmer, and cook for 10 minutes. Remove from the heat, cover, and let stand for 5 minutes or until the liquid has been absorbed. (See Kitchen Tip.)

4. PREPARE THE DRESSING AND DRESS THE SALAD In a large bowl, whisk together the oil, vinegar, mustard, honey, and salt and pepper to taste. Add the bulgur, Brussels sprouts, pomegranate arils, tangerine, green onion, and mint. Toss to mix, and serve at room temperature. Store leftover salad in an airtight container in the refrigerator and eat within 1 day.

KITCHEN TIP: You can prep the bulgur (step 3) in advance and store it in the refrigerator for up to 5 days. You can also cook more than you need for this recipe, adding in the extra to your weekly menu, so that it includes even more whole grains.

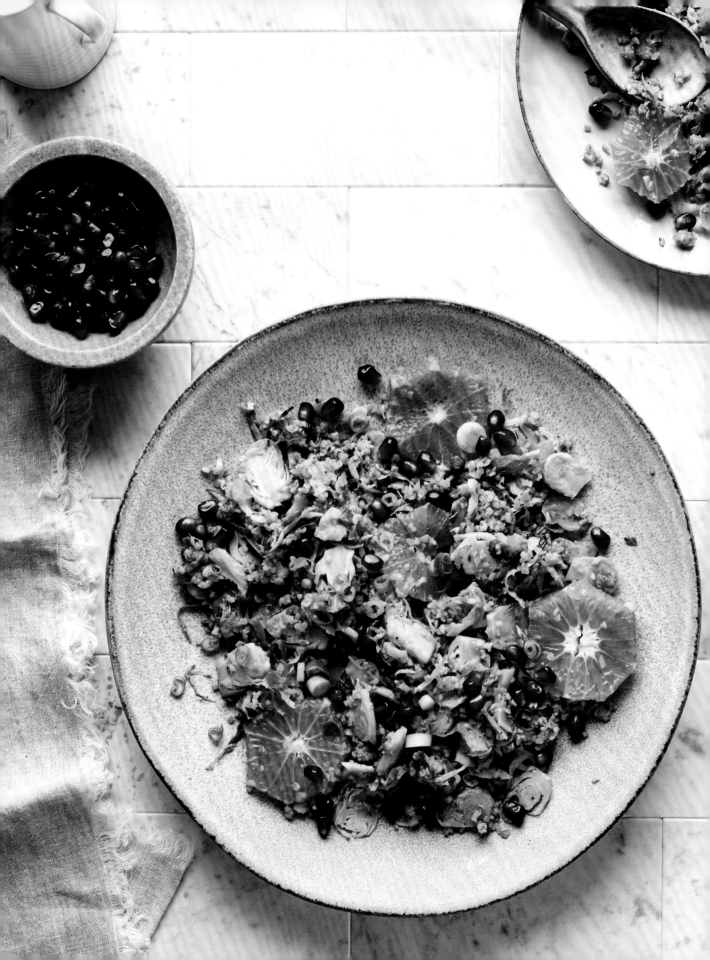

Everyday Green Salad

Vegetarian · Dairy-free · Gluten-free · Nut-free

My mother instilled in me the need to care for one's ingredients. Her weekly ritual of washing, drying, and meticulously storing her greens upon returning from the grocery store is the single most impactful habit I practice today (see Kitchen Tip). This salad, as simple as it may seem, is a way to enjoy fresh greens on a daily basis—a core nutritional principle of the Mediterranean diet. SERVES 4 TO 6

1 head romaine lettuce, chopped (about 6 cups/1.5 L) (see Kitchen Tip)

2 cups (500 mL) packed arugula

½ head radicchio, thinly sliced

½ fennel bulb, thinly sliced

6 radishes, thinly sliced

Everyday Dressing (page 246)

1. In a large bowl, combine the lettuce, arugula, radicchio, fennel, and radishes. Drizzle with the dressing, toss to mix, and serve.

KITCHEN TIP: Once your lettuce leaves are rinsed and spun dry, roll them in a clean kitchen towel, tuck them in a resealable bag, and store in the refrigerator. You will have fresh greens at the ready that will last for up to 1 week—certainly longer than pre-washed grocery store versions.

Spicy Broccoli Rice with Parmesan

Vegetarian • Gluten-free • Nut-free

I love broccoli, but my family does not have the same fondness for it. It used to be a tough sell to my small children and husband alike, which was unfortunate because I tried to eat it regularly. That's because cruciferous vegetables contain unique sulfur compounds known for their anti-inflammatory properties. But when the broccoli is prepared this way, the whole family asks for extra helpings. I tame back the chili for the kids, but the extra kick is part of what makes this side dish so addictive, so I keep it in for the adults. Serve this as a side dish, or topped with a runny poached egg and parmesan shavings for a delicious lunch. SERVES 4

1. In a food processor fitted with a steel blade, pulse the broccoli until it resembles rice, about 5 to 10 pulses. Work in batches so as not to overcrowd the machine. From the pulsed broccoli, measure out 3 cups (750 mL) broccoli rice (see Nutrition Note).

2. Heat the oil in a 12-inch (30 cm) non-stick skillet set over medium heat. Add the onion and sauté for 5 minutes or until softened. Add the garlic and chili flakes and cook for 1 minute or until fragrant.

3. Add the broccoli rice and salt and pepper to taste. Sauté for 5 minutes or until softened. Finally, add the parmesan, stir to combine, remove from the heat, and serve. Any leftovers can be stored in an airtight container in the refrigerator for up to 3 days.

1 head broccoli, chopped into small florets (see Nutrition Note)

2 Tbsp (30 mL) olive oil

1 large Vidalia onion, finely chopped

2 cloves garlic, minced

¼ tsp (1 mL) chili flakes

Salt and pepper

½ cup (125 mL) freshly grated Parmigiano Reggiano

NUTRITION NOTE: Any additional shredded broccoli can be enjoyed raw sprinkled over salads or added to soup or stir-fries—an easy way to increase the veg factor of a meal.

Orzo with Roasted Cauliflower, Raisins, and Pine Nuts

Vegan • Vegetarian • Dairy-free

I love pine nuts. They have a delicate flavor and a buttery yet crunchy texture, and they add a dose of heart-healthy fat and fiber to dishes, like this sweet and savory side. That said, pine nuts are fairly expensive, so feel free to use sliced almonds in this recipe instead. I like to serve this flavorful orzo alongside simple grilled fish or poultry marinated in a Lemon and Herb Marinade (page 247). SERVES 4 TO 6

1 cauliflower, cut into 1½-inch (4 cm) florets (about 8 cups/2 L)

2 shallots, sliced

3 Tbsp (45 mL) olive oil, divided

Salt and pepper

1 cup (250 mL) orzo

¼ cup (60 mL) pine nuts

¼ cup (60 mL) raisins

Zest of 1 lemon

½ cup (125 mL) chopped fresh flat-leaf parsley

1. Preheat the oven to 425°F (220°C). Line a baking sheet with parchment paper.

2. Place the cauliflower and shallots in a large bowl. Drizzle with 1 Tbsp (15 mL) olive oil, just enough to coat. Season with salt and pepper, toss, and spread evenly on the prepared baking sheet. Bake for about 20 minutes, tossing halfway through, until the cauliflower is golden brown.

3. Meanwhile, bring a saucepan of salted water to a boil. Add the orzo and cook according to the package directions. Drain.

4. Place the pine nuts in a small, dry skillet and toast until fragrant, 2 to 3 minutes. Be careful not to brown them too much.

5. In a large bowl, place the cooked orzo, the remaining 2 Tbsp (30 mL) oil, roasted cauliflower, pine nuts, raisins, lemon zest, and parsley. Toss and serve at room temperature. Any leftovers can be stored in an airtight container in the refrigerator for up to 2 days.

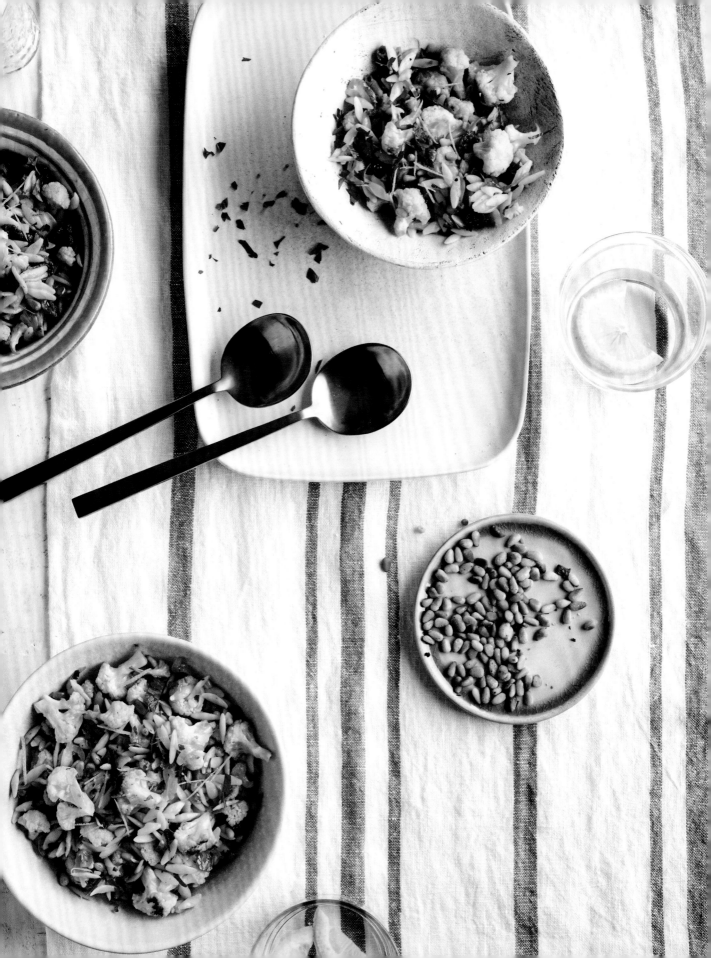

Greek Stuffed Tomatoes

Vegetarian • Nut-free

Most modern recipes for stuffed vegetables include a form of minced meat. Because red meat is eaten fairly infrequently in the Mediterranean diet, bread is commonly used as the main stuffing ingredient. Whole grain sourdough, olives, feta, and oregano are packed into juicy tomatoes to create a bite reminiscent of a Greek salad, yet warming and full of flavor. SERVES 6

6 vine tomatoes

2 tsp (10 mL) olive oil, plus more for drizzling

½ onion, diced

2 slices of whole grain sourdough bread, crusts removed and cubed

½ cup (125 mL) crumbled feta

¼ cup (60 mL) sliced Kalamata olives

¼ cup (60 mL) chopped fresh flat-leaf parsley

1 Tbsp (15 mL) fresh oregano

Pepper

1. Preheat the oven to 375°F (190°C).

2. Trim the tops off the tomatoes and hollow the inside using a spoon. Place them in a baking dish and set them aside.

3. Heat the oil in an 8-inch (20 cm) non-stick pan set over medium-high heat. Add the onion and cook for 5 minutes or until softened. Transfer to a bowl and let cool slightly.

4. Add the bread, feta, olives, parsley, and oregano to the cooled onion. Add pepper to taste and stir to combine.

5. Stuff the hollowed-out tomatoes with the filling. Drizzle the top with oil and bake for 25 to 30 minutes, until the stuffing is golden brown. Serve hot or at room temperature.

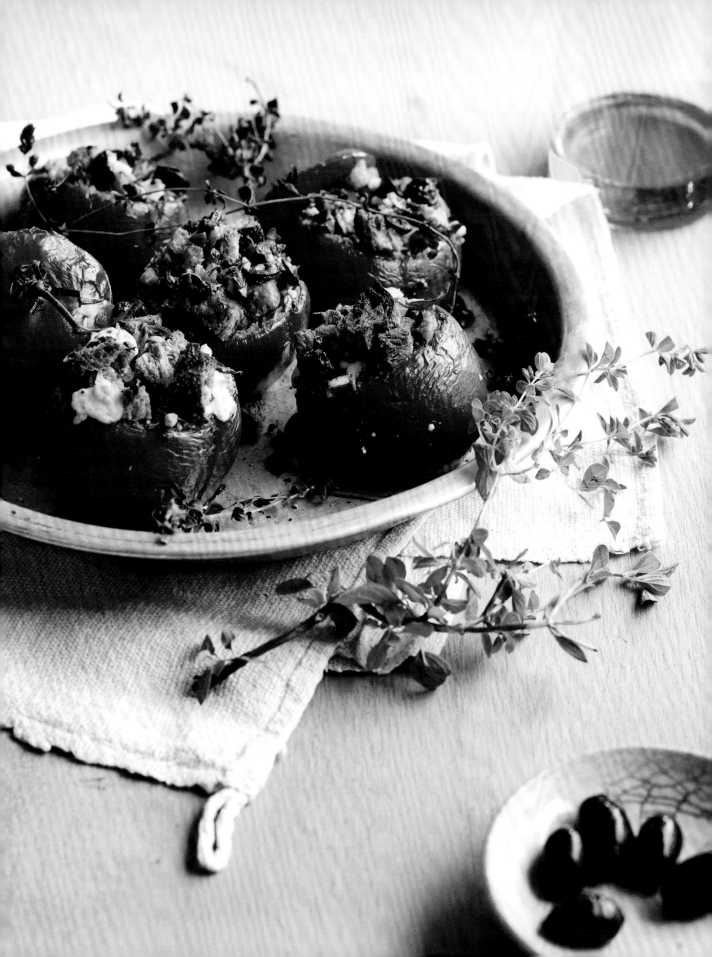

Smashed Potatoes with Garlic, Paprika, and Thyme

Vegan • Vegetarian • Dairy-free • Gluten-free • Nut-free

The humble potato doesn't get enough nutritional praise, in my honest opinion. Potatoes are inexpensive and pantry-friendly, and they contribute key nutrients to our diets, including vitamin C, potassium, and fiber. (Just remember to keep the skin on to get the full fiber benefit!) This dish showcases one of my favorite techniques for enjoying the whole potato, creating a crispy, snappy exterior and a tender center. The potatoes are brushed in a flavorful paprika and thyme oil that transforms them into a standout side dish.

SERVES 6 TO 8

2 lb (1 kg) fingerling potatoes, scrubbed (see Kitchen Tip)

3 Tbsp (45 mL) olive oil

3 garlic cloves, minced

1 tsp (5 mL) paprika

4 sprigs of thyme

Salt and pepper

1. Preheat the oven to 425°F (220°C) (use convection setting or for further advice, see page 61).

2. Place the potatoes in a large pot, cover with cold water, and add a generous pinch of salt. Bring to a boil, then simmer for 20 minutes or until tender. Drain and transfer to a baking sheet.

3. Using the bottom of a glass, press firmly on each potato to flatten to a ½ inch (1.2 cm) thickness.

4. In an 8-inch (20 cm) non-stick skillet set over medium-low heat, place the oil, garlic, paprika, and thyme, and allow the mixture to infuse, 3 to 5 minutes. Remove from the heat and brush over the potatoes, getting into every nook. Season with salt and pepper.

5. Bake for 20 minutes or until the potatoes are golden brown. Any leftovers can be stored in an airtight container in the refrigerator for up to 2 days. Reheat in an oven preheated to 425°F (220°C) for 5 to 10 minutes.

KITCHEN TIP: Fingerling potatoes, small and elongated, have a meaty, silky, and slightly sweet flavor. They can be replaced by new potatoes in this recipe, if you like.

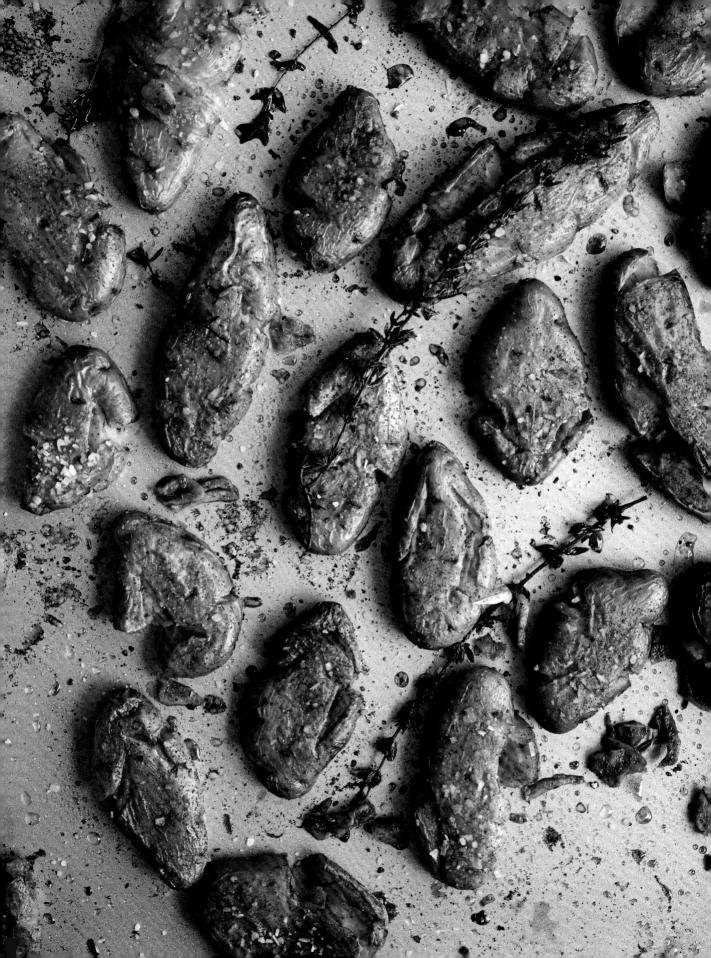

Grilled Zucchini with Minted Labneh and Pistachios

Vegetarian • Gluten-free

Zucchini are a kid-friendly vegetable because of their mild flavor, but for this same reason creativity is required to make them into a standout dish. In this side dish, the zucchini are first grilled for smokiness, then laid atop creamy labneh and topped with crunchy pistachios. Labneh, with a flavor that's a cross between yogurt and cream cheese, has become a mainstay in my refrigerator. It's tangy and creamy and here helps elevate the grilled zucchini. This makes for a stunning vegetable side for gatherings.

SERVES 4 TO 6

FOR THE LABNEH

½ cup (125 mL) labneh

2 Tbsp (30 mL) chopped fresh mint

Zest and juice of ½ lemon

Olive oil

FOR THE ZUCCHINI

4 zucchini, sliced lengthwise into ½-inch-thick (1.2 cm) slices

1 Tbsp (15 mL) olive oil

Salt and pepper

1 tsp (5 mL) za'atar, store-bought or homemade (page 245)

¼ cup (60 mL) pistachios, toasted and coarsely chopped

1. **PREPARE THE LABNEH** In a small bowl, combine the labneh, mint, lemon zest, and lemon juice. Spread on a serving platter, garnish with a drizzle of olive oil, and set aside.

2. Preheat the barbecue or a grill pan to medium-high and oil the grates.

3. **PREPARE THE ZUCCHINI** In a large bowl, toss the zucchini with the oil and season with salt and pepper. Make sure the zucchini are well coated and glossy. Grill the zucchini for 3 to 4 minutes per side.

4. Place the grilled zucchini on the labneh, sprinkle with the za'atar, and garnish with the pistachios.

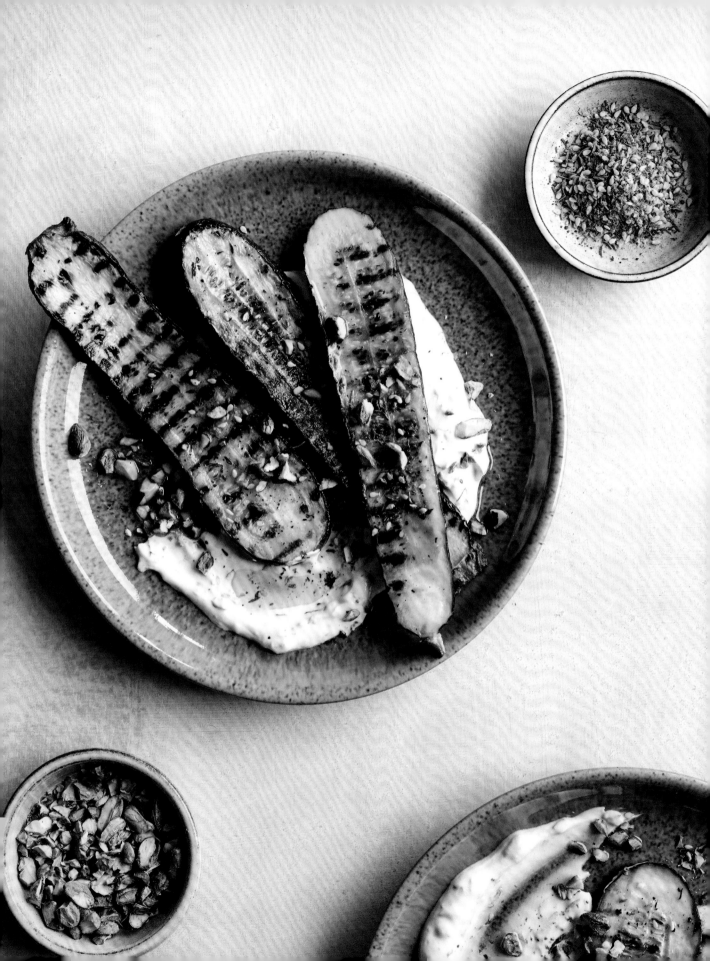

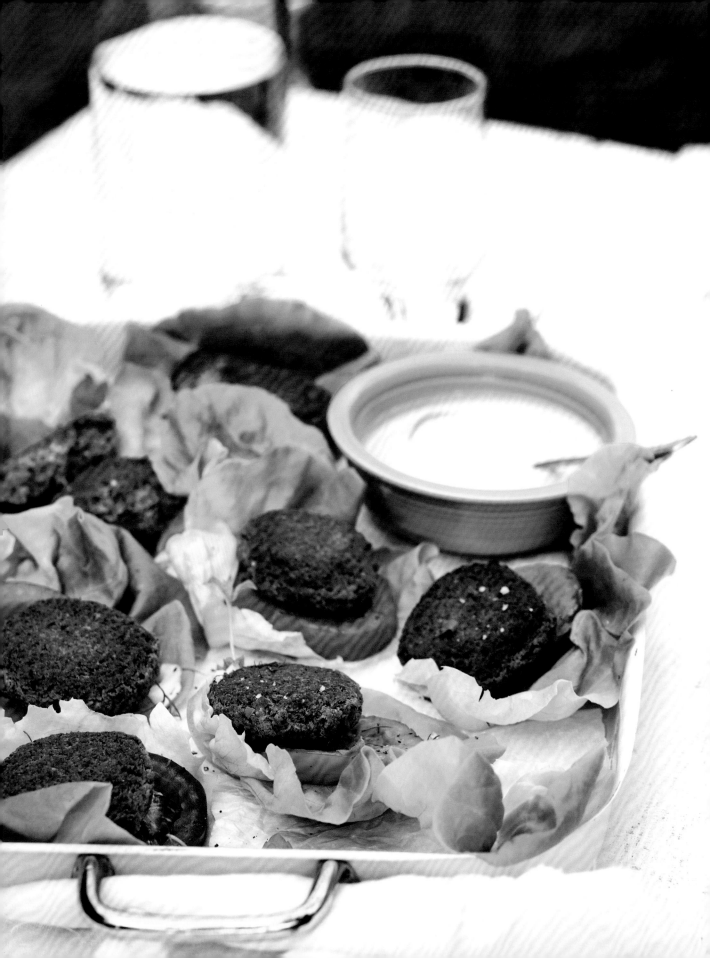

Vegetarian

Pulses are a staple of the Mediterranean eating pattern for their affordability and nutrition. Their fiber and protein help keep us fuller longer—and keep energy levels on an even keel. In this chapter, plant-based powerhouses—including lentils, beans, and chickpeas—shine, to help you work toward incorporating more vegetable-forward meals into your daily routine.

Mediterranean Farro and Chickpea Bowl

Vegetarian · Nut-free

This bowl works wonderfully for weekly lunches. It contains just the right balance of protein (from chickpeas), fiber (from veggies and grains), and fat (from the olive oil dressing) to keep you feeling full and energized for hours. The components are simple to prep in advance, and the flavors will have you looking forward to your midday break. If you don't have farro for this bowl, you can substitute 2 cups (500 mL) cooked brown rice.

SERVES 4 TO 6

1 cup (250 mL) farro, rinsed

3 cups (750 mL) water

1 bay leaf

Pinch of salt

1 onion, minced

2 garlic cloves, crushed

1 yellow bell pepper, sliced

1 red bell pepper, sliced

1 zucchini, sliced

Olive oil

1 can (19 oz/540 mL) chickpeas, drained and rinsed

½ cup (125 mL) Balsamic Vinaigrette (page 246)

⅓ cup (80 mL) crumbled feta

1 cup (250 mL) arugula, radish, or sunflower microgreens (see Nutrition Note)

1. In a saucepan, bring the farro, water, bay leaf, and salt to a boil, reduce to a simmer, and cook, uncovered, for 25 to 30 minutes, until the farro is al dente. Drain.

2. Preheat the oven to 400°F (200°C). Line a baking sheet with parchment paper.

3. In a large bowl, toss the onion, garlic, bell peppers, and zucchini with a drizzle of olive oil and salt to taste. Spread evenly on the prepared baking sheet. Roast for 35 to 40 minutes, turning halfway through, until the vegetables are tender and their edges are caramelized.

4. Divide the farro, roasted vegetables, and chickpeas among individual bowls. Drizzle with the vinaigrette and top with the feta and microgreens.

NUTRITION NOTE: Did you know that microgreens are just as nutritious as their mature counterparts? Use them to enhance your salads, sandwiches, or even avocado toast (like the one on page 78). Pea, mustard, and radish sprouts all pack a nutritional punch and come with tons of flavor to boot.

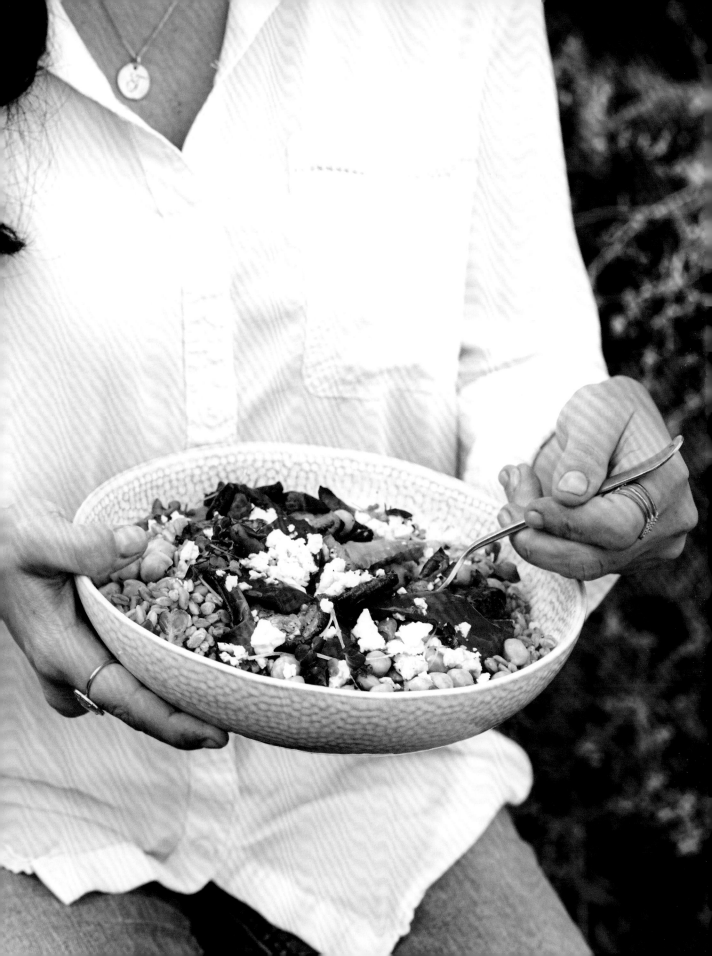

Eggplant Polpette

Vegetarian • Nut-free

Inspired by the traditional Calabrian dish, these eggplant polpette are a surprisingly meaty, tender, and flavorful vegetarian alternative. Serve these as you would traditional meatballs, alongside spaghetti or other pasta, or at your next dinner party as an appetizer that will have everyone singing its praises. SERVES 4 TO 6

1 Tbsp (15 mL) olive oil

1 large or 2 small eggplant, diced (about 5 cups/1.25 L)

Salt and pepper

1 cup (250 mL) plain breadcrumbs, store-bought (like panko) or homemade (page 244)

2 eggs, lightly beaten

⅓ cup (80 mL) grated Pecorino Romano, plus more to garnish

1 garlic clove, minced

½ cup (125 mL) finely chopped fresh flat-leaf parsley

2 cups (500 mL) marinara sauce, store-bought or homemade (page 248)

½ cup (125 mL) fresh basil

1. Preheat the oven to 400°F (200°C) (use convection setting or for further advice, see page 61). Grease a baking sheet with enough olive oil so that it is evenly glossy.

2. Heat the oil in a 12-inch (30 cm) non-stick skillet set over medium heat. Add the eggplant and salt and pepper to taste and sauté for 10 to 15 minutes, until very tender. Transfer the eggplant to a large bowl and mash using a potato masher to a coarse purée.

3. Add the breadcrumbs, eggs, Pecorino, garlic, and parsley. Season with salt and pepper and mix well.

4. Using a 2 Tbsp (30 mL) measuring scoop, form the mixture into balls, and place on the prepared baking sheet.

5. Bake for 20 minutes, gently turning halfway through, until the polpette are nice golden brown on both sides. Meanwhile, heat the sauce in a saucepan.

6. Place the polpette in a serving dish and top with the warm sauce. Garnish with the basil and a sprinkle of Pecorino.

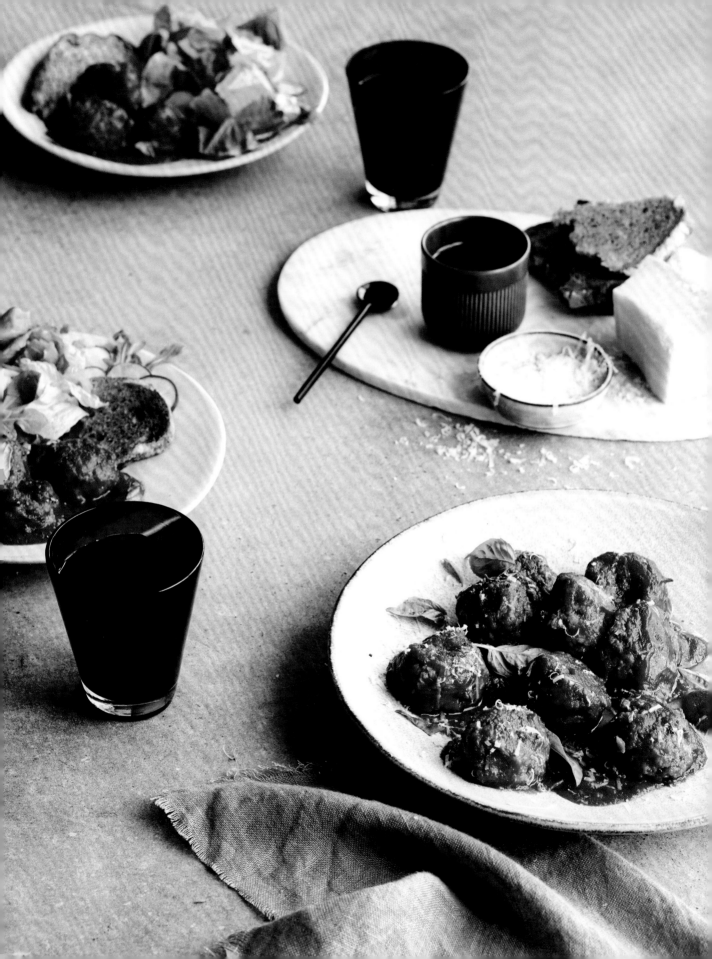

Garlicky Rapini Galette

Vegetarian • Nut-free

Bitter greens hold a special place in the Mediterranean diet. Foraged almost daily, bitter greens are typically served with a generous glug of olive oil, on the side at lunch and dinner. Although these greens are nutritionally beneficial and touted as digestive aids, many people struggle with the bitter flavor. This recipe takes the traditional preparation of bitter greens one step further, tucking them into a rustic tart designed to make its star ingredient shine. The combination of flakey crust and sharp garlic is ideal for showcasing the rapini. SERVES 6

FOR THE CRUST

1¼ cups (310 mL) spelt or all-purpose flour

½ cup (125 mL) cold unsalted butter, diced

½ tsp (2.5 mL) kosher salt

2 to 3 Tbsp (30 to 45 mL) ice water

FOR THE FILLING

2 bunches of rapini (broccoli rabe), ends trimmed

2 Tbsp (30 mL) olive oil

5 garlic cloves, sliced

¼ tsp (1 mL) crushed chili flakes

Salt and pepper

½ cup (125 mL) grated provolone

TO FINISH

1 egg yolk, beaten

2 Tbsp (30 mL) grated Parmigiano Reggiano

1. **PREPARE THE CRUST** In a food processor fitted with a steel blade, pulse the flour, butter, and salt together until the mixture resembles small peas. With the motor running at low speed, pour in the water and process until the dough pulls away from the sides of the bowl.

2. Transfer the dough to a floured work surface. Form into a disc, wrap it in plastic wrap, and place it in the refrigerator to chill for at least 1 hour.

3. Preheat the oven to 350°F (180°C).

4. **PREPARE THE FILLING** Bring a large pot of salted water to a boil. Add the rapini and cook for 3 minutes, then drain well.

5. Heat the oil in a 12-inch (30 cm) non-stick skillet set over medium heat. Add the garlic and chili flakes, and cook until fragrant, 1 minute. Add the rapini and sauté for 2 to 3 minutes, until well coated in the seasoned oil. Season with salt and pepper, remove from the heat, and let cool (see Kitchen Tip).

6. Place a sheet of parchment paper on your work surface. Unwrap the chilled dough and place it on the parchment paper. Place another sheet of parchment on top of the dough, then roll it out to form a disc about 14 inches (35 cm) wide and ½ inch (1.2 cm) thick. Remove the top sheet of parchment. Transfer the bottom piece of parchment with the dough on it to the baking sheet.

recipe continues

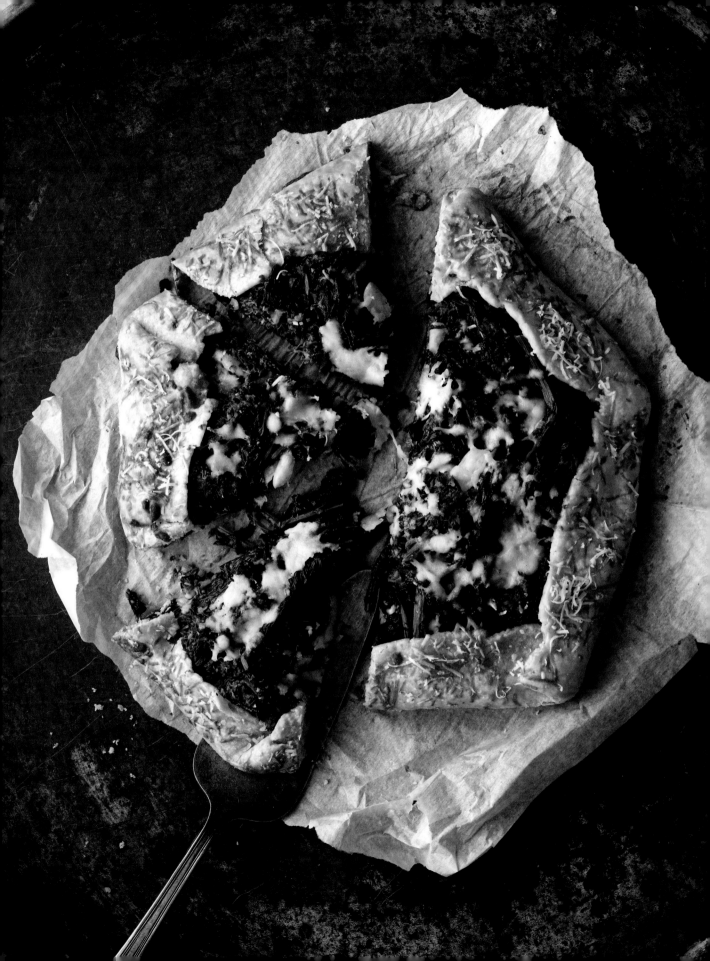

7. Place the sautéed rapini in the center of the dough disc, leaving a 1-inch (2.5 cm) border all around. Fold the exposed edge of dough in toward the center, partially enclosing the filling. Top the rapini with the provolone. Brush the sides of the galette with the egg yolk and sprinkle with the parmesan.

8. Bake for 35 minutes or until the crust is golden brown. Serve at room temperature.

KITCHEN TIP: You can cook your rapini ahead of time. It will keep in the refrigerator, stored in an airtight container, for up to 3 days.

Sumac Bean Salad

Vegan • Vegetarian • Dairy-free • Gluten-free • Nut-free

If I'm so keen on canned beans and chickpeas, it's because they turn a salad into a balanced meal in less than a minute. Here, herbs and spices—key flavor enhancers in the Mediterranean diet—are the secret to bringing the hearty beans to life. Mint and parsley add a wisp of freshness, while the tangy sumac dressing adds brightness, making it perfect for the lunch box. SERVES 4 TO 6

1. **PREPARE THE SALAD** In a large bowl, toss together the black beans, chickpeas, cucumbers, tomatoes, olives, mint, and parsley.

2. **MAKE THE VINAIGRETTE** In a small bowl, whisk together the mustard, shallots, lemon juice, and sumac. Pour in the olive oil in an even stream while whisking to emulsify.

3. Pour the dressing over the salad. Toss well, season with salt and pepper, and serve. Any leftovers can be stored in an airtight container in the refrigerator for up to 2 days.

FOR THE SALAD

1 can (19 oz/540 mL) black beans, drained and rinsed

1 can (19 oz/540 mL) chickpeas, drained and rinsed

2 Persian cucumbers, diced

2 Roma tomatoes, cored and diced

½ cup (125 mL) sliced green olives

¼ cup (60 mL) chopped fresh mint

¼ cup (60 mL) chopped fresh flat-leaf parsley

FOR THE VINAIGRETTE

1 tsp (5 mL) Dijon mustard

2 shallots, minced

Juice of ½ lemon

2 tsp (10 mL) sumac

¼ cup (60 mL) extra virgin olive oil

Salt and pepper

Moroccan Squash and Chickpea Stew

Vegetarian • Dairy-free • Gluten-free • Nut-free

This stew has become an autumn staple in my household, as it showcases one of my favorite vegetables, the butternut squash. Simmered with high-protein chickpeas and warming spices, this meal hits sweet, savory, and spicy notes all at once. It is a complete meal on its own and freezes beautifully, but you can also serve this alongside rice, to soak up some of the stew's flavorful juices. SERVES 6

1 Tbsp (15 mL) olive oil

2 cups (500 mL) diced onion

2 red bell peppers, diced

2 garlic cloves, minced

1 Tbsp (15 mL) paprika

1 tsp (5 mL) ground cumin

½ tsp (2.5 mL) ground coriander

½ tsp (2.5 mL) ground ginger

1 butternut squash, peeled and cut into 1-inch (2.5 cm) cubes (about 6 cups/1.5 L)

1 can (19 oz/540 mL) chickpeas, drained and rinsed

1 can (14 oz/398 mL) diced tomatoes

1 Tbsp (15 mL) honey

4 cups (1 L) vegetable broth

Salt and pepper

2 cups (500 mL) frozen chopped spinach

1. Heat the oil in a large pot set over medium-high heat. Add the onion and peppers, and cook for 5 minutes or until the vegetables have softened.

2. Stir in the garlic, paprika, cumin, coriander, and ginger, and cook for 1 minute, until fragrant (see Kitchen Tip).

3. Add the squash, chickpeas, tomatoes, and honey. Pour in the broth. Season with salt and pepper, stir, and then bring to a boil. Simmer for 20 minutes or until the squash is tender.

4. Adjust the seasoning to taste, add the spinach, and cook for 5 minutes or until wilted. Serve. Any leftovers can be stored in an airtight container in the refrigerator for up to 3 days or in the freezer for up to 3 months.

KITCHEN TIP: To get the most flavor from your spices, cook them along with the oil, onion, and bell pepper. Since the main aromatic compounds are fat soluble (they dissolve in fat), this step will create a more complex flavor base.

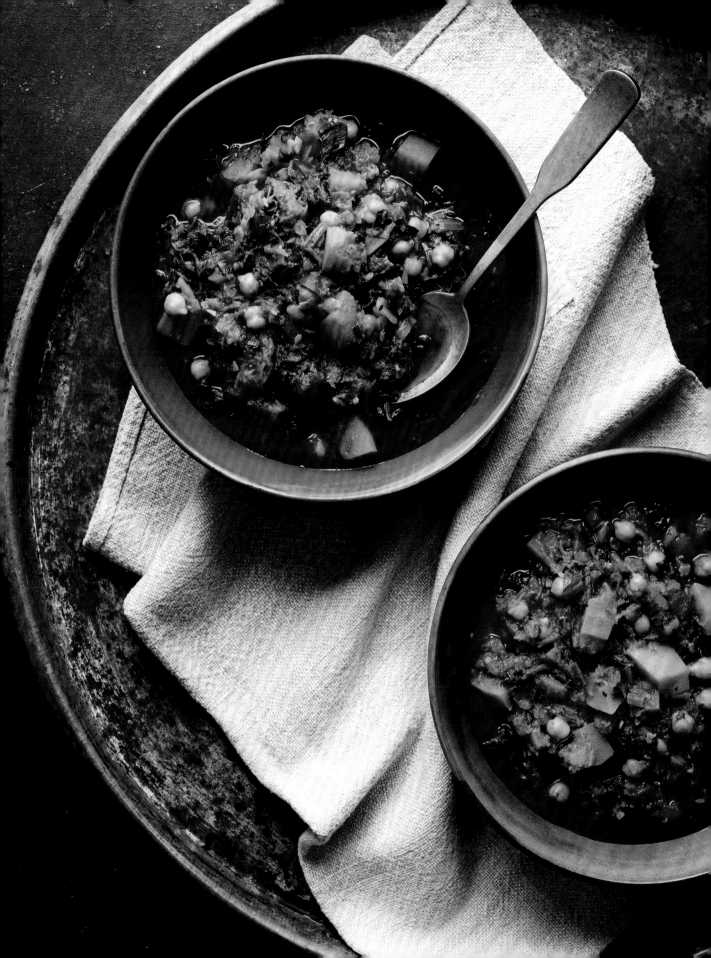

Oven-Baked Spinach Falafel

Vegan · Vegetarian · Dairy-free · Gluten-free · Nut-free

Bright green and full of flavor, these herb-filled patties are surprisingly simple to prepare. Unlike the traditional deep-fried falafel, these patties are oven-baked—the trick to creating a crisp exterior being a well-oiled baking sheet. It's important to use dried chickpeas in this recipe to obtain the right texture, so you'll want to plan ahead for the soaking step. I like to serve these falafel in crisp lettuce wraps, drizzled with tahini sauce, though they can very well be served on their own, with the tahini sauce on the side for dipping. During the week, I tend to toss any leftovers into a salad for a hit of plant-based protein.

MAKES 12 FALAFEL

1 cup (250 mL) dried chickpeas

2 garlic cloves, halved

1 small onion, chopped (about ½ cup/125 mL)

½ cup (125 mL) frozen chopped spinach, thawed and pressed of excess water

½ cup (125 mL) fresh flat-leaf parsley

¼ cup (60 mL) fresh dill

1 tsp (5 mL) ground cumin

½ tsp (2.5 mL) ground coriander

¼ tsp (1 mL) ground turmeric

¼ tsp (1 mL) cayenne pepper

½ tsp (2.5 mL) baking powder

Salt and pepper

TO SERVE (OPTIONAL)

1 head butter lettuce, leaves pulled apart

1 tomato, sliced

Fresh mint

Tahini Sauce (page 249)

1. Place the chickpeas in a large bowl and cover with cold water by at least 2 inches (5 cm). Let soak for 8 hours or overnight. Drain.

2. Preheat the oven to 400°F (200°C) (use convection setting or for further advice, see page 61). Grease a baking sheet with oil.

3. In a food processor fitted with a steel blade, process the chickpeas for 2 minutes, scraping down the sides of the bowl from time to time. The mixture should stick between your fingers.

4. Add the garlic, onion, spinach, parsley, dill, cumin, coriander, turmeric, cayenne pepper, baking powder, and salt and pepper to taste. Process until smooth.

5. Using a 2 Tbsp (30 mL) measuring scoop, form the mixture into small patties, and place on the prepared baking sheet.

6. Bake for 26 to 28 minutes, turning halfway through, until they are golden brown.

7. Enjoy in lettuce cups with tomato, mint, and a drizzle of tahini sauce, or on their own, served with the tahini sauce for dipping. Any leftovers can be stored in an airtight container in the refrigerator for up to 3 days. Reheat in the oven at 400°F (200°C) for 7 minutes or until warmed through. They also freeze very well: cool completely, then store in an airtight container for up to 3 months.

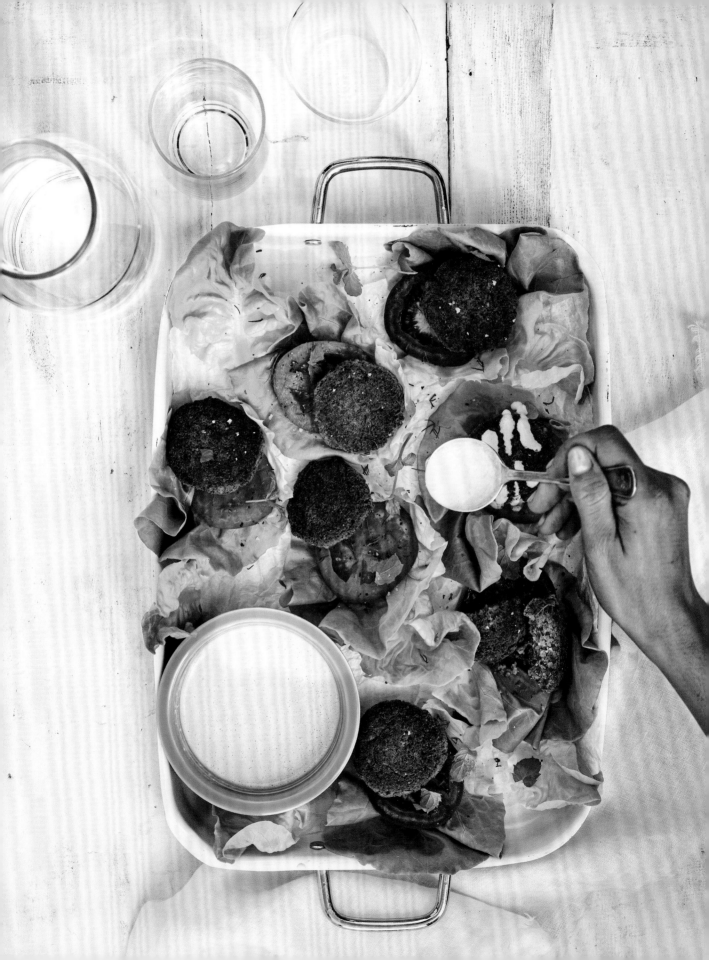

Zucchini and Ricotta Sformato

Vegetarian • Gluten-free • Nut-free

Zucchini flowers are the ultimate summer delicacy. Their harvesting window being small, I'm always looking for ways to make the most of their short season. They're typically stuffed and fried (and delicious!), but I like adding them to the top of this sformato (part flan, part frittata), as you get to appreciate their delicate flavor, which naturally goes well with the zucchini-loaded custard. Out of season, you can prepare this recipe and omit the decorative flowers, for an equally delicious dish that's a lovely make-ahead brunch option.

SERVES 6

2 tsp (10 mL) olive oil

1 onion, finely diced

2 zucchini, thinly sliced

1 tub (16 oz/475 g) ricotta

4 eggs, beaten

¼ cup (60 mL) chopped fresh flat-leaf parsley

3 Tbsp (45 mL) freshly grated Pecorino Romano

Salt and pepper

10 zucchini flowers, stamen removed

1. Preheat the oven to 350°F (180°C). Grease a 10-inch (25 cm) springform pan with oil.

2. Heat the oil in a 10-inch (25 cm) non-stick skillet set over medium heat. Add the onion and sauté for 5 minutes or until softened. Add the zucchini and cook for 2 minutes or until softened. Remove from the heat and let cool slightly.

3. In a large bowl and using a fork, mix together the ricotta and eggs until smooth. Add the parsley, Pecorino, and cooked zucchini mixture. Season with salt and pepper, and stir to combine.

4. Pour the mixture into the prepared pan. Fan the zucchini flowers on the surface, pressing them into the mixture slightly.

5. Bake for 55 minutes or until the center of the sformato is no longer jiggly and the edges are golden brown. Let cool before unmolding, and serve at room temperature.

KITCHEN TIP: Frittatas and variants such as this one are commonly served at room temperature. This can be made ahead and brought to room temperature to serve when guests arrive.

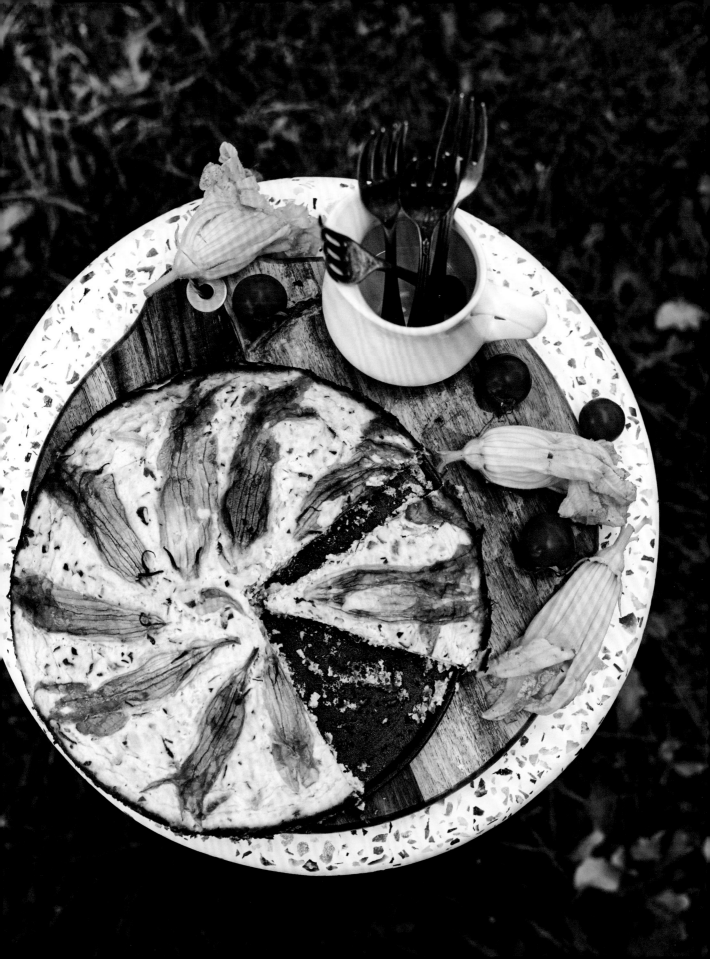

Bolognese with Lentils and Mushrooms

Vegan • Vegetarian • Dairy-free • Gluten-free • Nut-free

This plant-based sauce gets its sustenance from protein-packed lentils, while mushrooms lend a depth of flavor reminiscent of meat. Serve over pasta, such as pappardelle, or, for even more veggies, along with roasted spaghetti squash. SERVES 4 TO 6

1 package (½ oz/15 g) dried wild mushrooms

1 cup (250 mL) boiling water

1 onion, quartered

1 celery stalk, cut into chunks

1 carrot, peeled and cut into chunks

1 package (8 oz/227 g) cremini mushrooms

2 garlic cloves

2 Tbsp (30 mL) olive oil

1 Tbsp (15 mL) tomato paste

1 cup (250 mL) French (Puy) lentils

1 jar (24 oz/680 mL) tomato purée (passata)

1 sprig of thyme

½ cup (125 mL) fresh basil

4 cups (1 L) water

Salt and pepper

1. Soak the dried mushrooms in the boiling water for at least 5 minutes. Set aside, reserving the soaking liquid.

2. In a food processor fitted with a steel blade, process the onion, celery, carrot, cremini mushrooms, and garlic into a coarse meal (see Kitchen Tip).

3. Set a large pot over medium heat and add the oil. Add the processed vegetables, and sauté for 5 minutes or until softened. Stir in the tomato paste, ensuring the vegetables are evenly coated, and cook for 1 minute. Add the rehydrated mushrooms and their soaking water, along with the lentils, tomato purée, thyme, basil, water, and salt and pepper to taste. Stir, then bring to a boil.

4. Reduce the heat to medium-low, cover partially, and simmer for 30 minutes or until the lentils are tender. Adjust the seasoning to taste and serve. Any leftovers can be stored in an airtight container in the refrigerator for up to 3 days or in the freezer for up to 3 months.

KITCHEN TIP: The food processor saves a lot of time when preparing this sauce. Coarsely processing the vegetables also helps them blend right in with the lentils, giving the sauce a uniform texture. This trick works for any bolognese sauce, whether it's with meat or a vegetarian version.

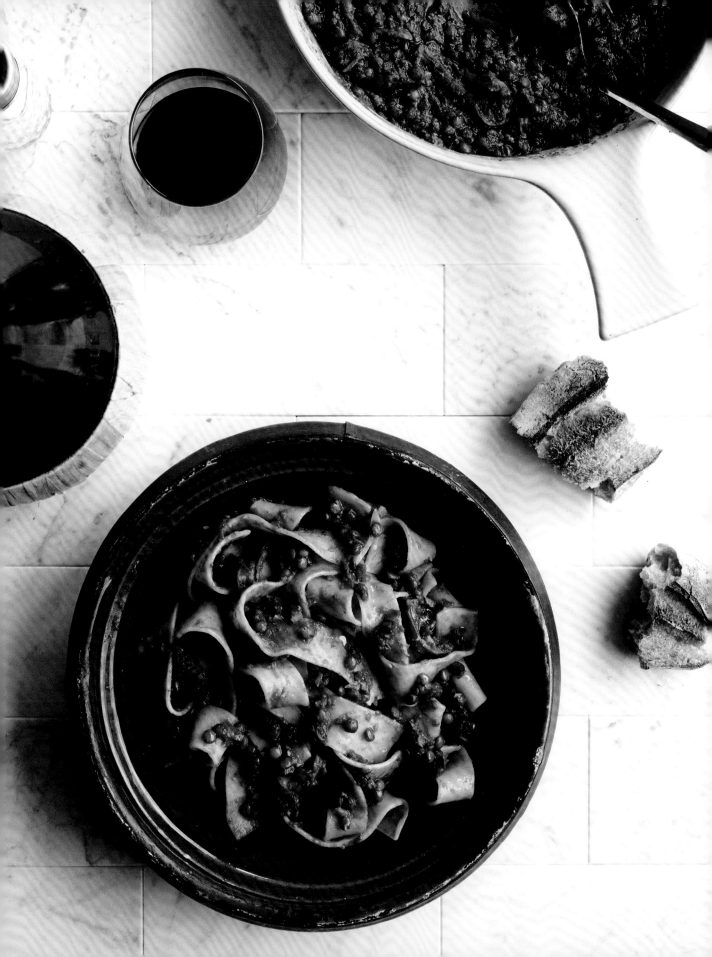

Creamy Farfalle Pasta Salad with Artichoke Hearts

Vegetarian • Nut-free

Artichokes are a classic ingredient in Mediterranean cuisine. They are rich in fiber, particularly the prebiotic kind, which is known to improve the growth of good bacteria in the gut. This recipe uses canned artichoke hearts, which not only are a time-saver but also easier on digestion (their high fiber content sometimes causes a little tummy turbulence). They pair wonderfully with this pasta salad's zesty avocado dressing, an herb-packed sauce that adds creaminess and healthy fat to the salad. The addition of protein-rich hemp seeds helps round off this dish so it may be eaten on its own for a weekday lunch, or as a side dish that will crush your next cookout. SERVES 4 TO 6

FOR THE SAUCE

1 ripe avocado

1½ cups (375 mL) fresh basil

¼ cup (60 mL) fresh mint

¼ cup (60 mL) hemp seeds

2 garlic cloves, minced

½ cup (125 mL) water

¼ cup (60 mL) olive oil

Juice of ½ lemon

Salt and pepper

FOR THE PASTA SALAD

2½ cups (625 mL) farfalle

1 can (14 oz/398 mL) artichoke hearts, drained and chopped

1 cup (250 mL) cherry tomatoes, halved

¼ cup (60 mL) grated Parmigiano Reggiano (see Kitchen Tip)

1. **PREPARE THE SAUCE** In a food processor fitted with a steel blade, place the avocado, basil, mint, hemp seeds, and garlic. With the motor running, pour in the water, oil, and lemon juice, and process until smooth. Season with salt and pepper.

2. **PREPARE THE PASTA SALAD** Bring a large pot of salted water to a boil. Add the pasta and cook according to the package directions. Drain and let cool to room temperature in a serving bowl.

3. Pour the sauce over the pasta and toss to coat. Add the artichoke hearts, tomatoes, and parmesan, stirring to mix. Serve at room temperature. Any leftovers can be stored in an airtight container in the refrigerator for up to 2 days.

KITCHEN TIP: For a dairy-free alternative, replace the parmesan with 2 Tbsp (30 mL) nutritional yeast.

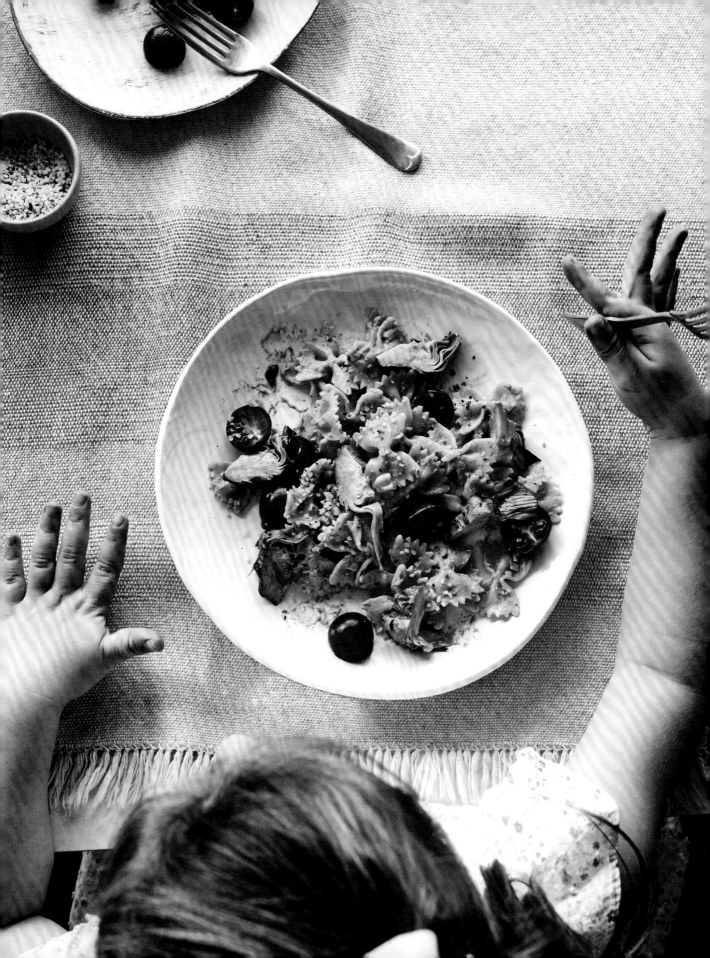

Dukkah-Crusted Whole Cauliflower

Vegan • Vegetarian • Dairy-free • Gluten-free

When my meat-loving husband saw the head of cauliflower on the dinner table, never did he imagine that he'd soon be smiling ear to ear, completely satisfied with his plant-based dinner. Fact is, with its 11 grams of protein and nearly 14 grams of fiber, it's no wonder a head of cauliflower makes for a filling main. Topped with a dukkah crust, it is absolutely delectable too. Dukkah is a fragrant mix of nuts, seeds (including sesame), and spices like cumin and coriander. In this recipe, the dukkah crusts the whole cauliflower, providing a burst of flavor with every floret. SERVES 4

½ cup (125 mL) almonds

2 Tbsp (30 mL) sesame seeds

1 Tbsp (15 mL) cumin seeds

1 Tbsp (15 mL) coriander seeds

½ tsp (2.5 mL) paprika

Salt

3 Tbsp (45 mL) olive oil

1 cauliflower (about 1½ lb/680 g) (see Kitchen Tip)

1 cup (250 mL) hummus, store-bought or homemade (pages 106–107)

1. In a small, dry skillet set over medium-high heat, toast the almonds, sesame seeds, cumin seeds, and coriander seeds until fragrant, 2 to 3 minutes. Transfer to a mortar and pestle (or food processor), add the paprika, and coarsely grind. Season with salt.

2. Transfer ½ cup (125 mL) of the dukkah to a bowl and add the oil. Mix into a paste and set aside. Store the leftover dukkah in an air-tight container at room temperature for up to 1 month.

3. Preheat the oven to 400°F (200°C). Line a baking sheet with parchment paper.

4. Trim the cauliflower leaves and stem so that the cauliflower sits upright. Place it in a large glass bowl with ¼ cup (60 mL) water and cook in the microwave on high power for 8 minutes.

5. Carefully transfer the cauliflower to the prepared baking sheet. Spread the dukkah over the cauliflower, tucking some of the mixture into the crevices as well. Bake for 35 to 40 minutes, until the top of the cauliflower is nicely browned.

6. Spread the hummus on a serving plate. Gently place the cauliflower on top of the hummus and serve.

KITCHEN TIP: Cauliflower leaves are a treat, so don't toss them! Cook them, lightly oiled, alongside the cauliflower on the baking sheet and enjoy.

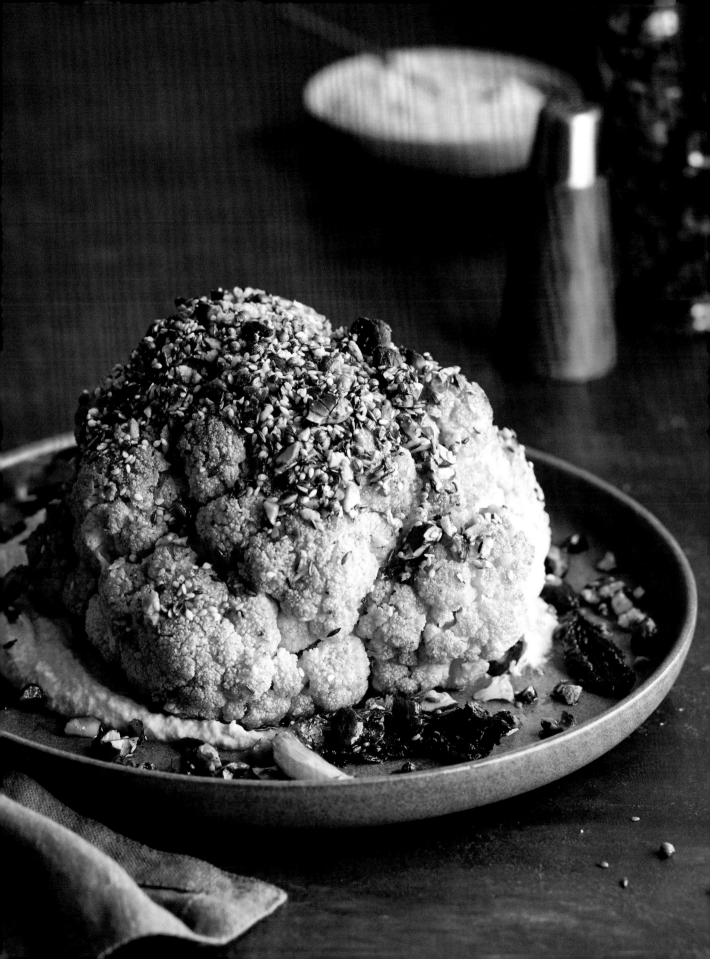

Creamy Asparagus Risotto

Vegetarian • Gluten-free • Nut-free

This classic risotto gets an elegant twist via the creamy asparagus sauce stirred in at the end of cooking. Fresh asparagus is first sautéed in olive oil, then puréed into a velvety sauce, adding a pop of color to the dish along with a healthy dose of folate and fiber. Serve this risotto in the spring when asparagus is in its prime. SERVES 4

3 Tbsp (45 mL) olive oil, divided

1 bunch of asparagus, ends trimmed, cut into 1-inch (2.5 cm) pieces (about 3 cups/750 mL)

Salt and pepper

5 cups (1.25 L) water or vegetable broth

1 onion, finely diced

1½ cups (375 mL) arborio or carnaroli rice

½ cup (125 mL) dry white wine

½ cup (125 mL) freshly grated Parmigiano Reggiano

¼ cup (60 mL) chopped fresh flat-leaf parsley

2 Tbsp (30 mL) salted butter

1. Heat 1 Tbsp (15 mL) oil in a large cast-iron or heavy-bottomed skillet set over medium-high heat. Add the asparagus and salt and pepper to taste, and toss. Pour in ¼ cup (60 mL) water, cover, and cook for 5 minutes or until tender but still bright green. Meanwhile, heat the water (or broth) in a small saucepan set over low heat.

2. Reserving a few asparagus tips for garnish, transfer the asparagus to a blender and purée until very smooth, adding 1 to 2 tsp (5 to 10 mL) olive oil to help smooth it out, if needed. Set aside.

3. In the same skillet, heat the remaining 2 Tbsp (30 mL) oil over medium-low heat. Add the onion and soften, 5 minutes, being careful not to brown it at this stage. Add the rice and, using a wooden spoon, stir to coat the grains well with the oil. Deglaze with the wine, stirring until it has evaporated.

4. Using a ladle, add ¾ cup (180 mL) of the warmed water (or broth) to the rice. Stir constantly, about 2 minutes, or until the liquid is almost all evaporated. Add another ladleful of liquid, repeating this step with the remaining water (or broth) until the rice is fully cooked but still firm to the bite—this process will take about 20 minutes. There should be some liquid left.

5. Stir in the asparagus purée, parmesan, and parsley. Stir in the butter and half a ladleful of liquid, then remove from the heat. Let stand for 5 minutes or until most of the liquid has absorbed and the consistency is creamy, not runny. Garnish with a few of the reserved asparagus tips and serve.

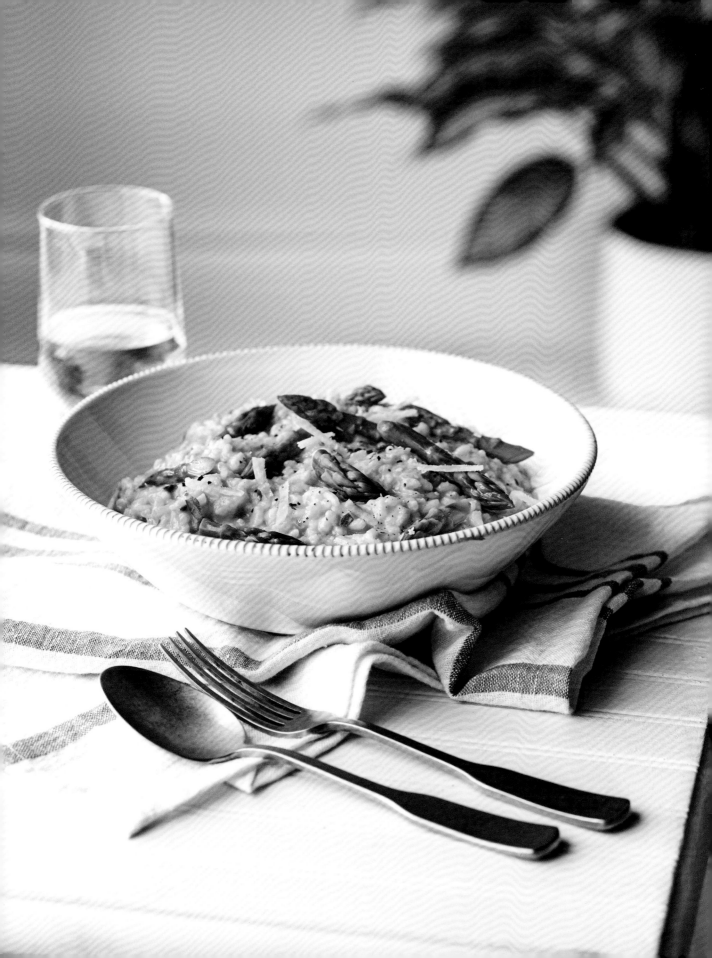

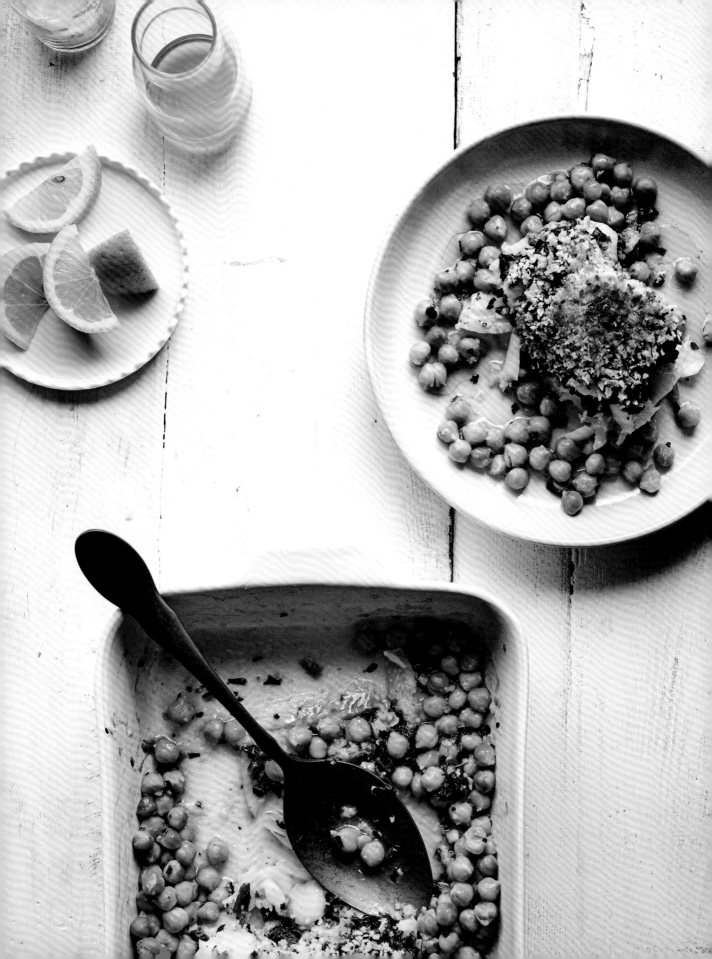

Fish and Seafood

In North America, many of us have the mistaken idea that fish and seafood are complicated to prepare, or should be reserved for special occasions. In reality, these ingredients are versatile and quick-cooking, never mind being highly nutritious and a regular part of the traditional Mediterranean diet. To inspire you, this chapter showcases fish and seafood in delicious ways, including simple yet elegant dishes like Baked Salmon with Gremolata Crust (page 182) and Mackerel Bucatini with Crispy Anchovy Breadcrumbs (page 176)—recipes designed to make a splash.

Saffron Rice with Shrimp and Chorizo

Dairy-free • Gluten-free • Nut-free

This is an ideal weeknight dinner, as it comes together quickly in just one pan. Saffron-scented rice creates the base for this paella-inspired dish; it's then loaded with smoky chorizo and protein-packed shrimp. Sweet peas and spinach add a pop of color and vegetables to the dish, making it a fully balanced meal with easy cleanup. Win-win. SERVES 6 TO 8

½ tsp (2.5 mL) saffron

2 Tbsp (30 mL) lukewarm water

2 Tbsp (30 mL) olive oil, divided

2 lb (1 kg) shrimp (size 31/40), peeled and deveined

½ lb (225 g) chorizo, cubed

2 tsp (10 mL) paprika

2 cups (500 mL) diced onion

4 garlic cloves, minced

1 Anaheim pepper or long sweet green pepper, finely chopped

½ cup (125 mL) dry white wine

1½ cups (375 mL) long-grain brown rice

3 cups (750 mL) no-salt-added chicken broth

Salt and pepper

1 cup (250 mL) frozen green peas

4 cups (1 L) packed baby spinach

1. In a small bowl, combine the saffron and water. Let infuse for at least 5 minutes.

2. Heat 1 Tbsp (15 mL) oil in a large Dutch oven set over medium-high heat. Add the shrimp, chorizo, and paprika, and brown for 3 minutes. Transfer to a plate.

3. In the same saucepan, heat the remaining 1 Tbsp (15 mL) oil over medium heat. Add the onion, garlic, and Anaheim pepper, and cook until softened, 3 minutes.

4. Deglaze with the wine, and allow it to reduce by half, about 2 minutes.

5. Pour in the rice, saffron with its soaking liquid, and broth. Season with salt and pepper, then bring to a boil. Reduce to low heat, cover, and cook for 15 minutes. Stir in the peas and spinach, then return the shrimp and chorizo to the pot. Cover and cook for 5 minutes or until the spinach is wilted and the shrimp is fully cooked through. Store in an airtight container in the refrigerator for up to 2 days.

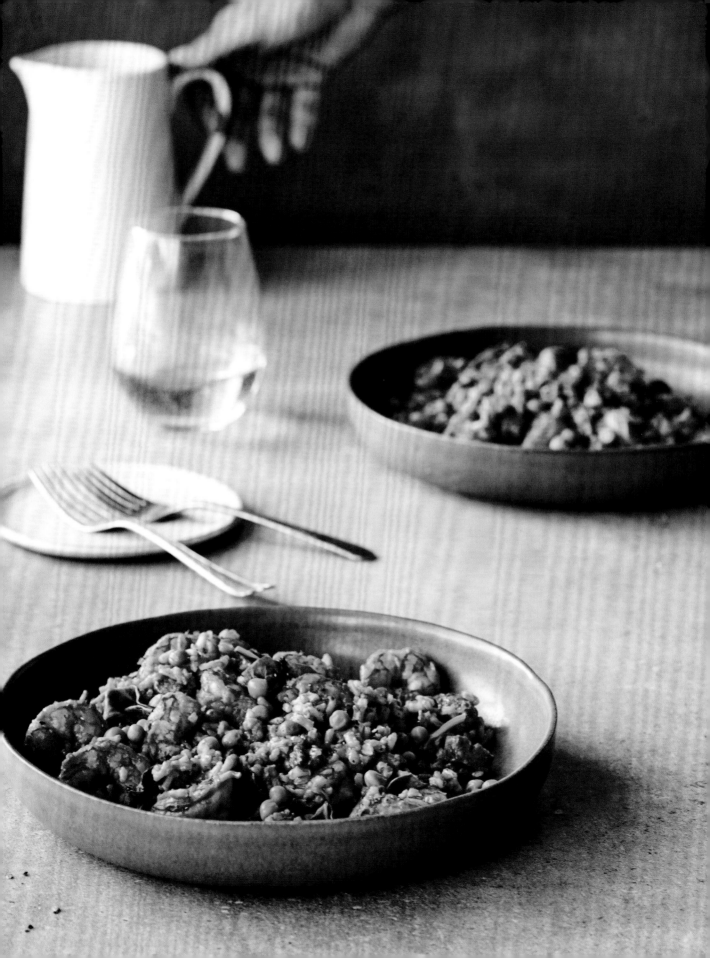

Cod, Spinach, and Chickpea Casserole

Vegetarian • Nut-free

If you're ever at a loss for what to make with cod, this casserole is for you. It has been on my winter rotation for years because of how simple and comforting it is. Layers of cod, sautéed spinach, and breadcrumbs result in a flavorful and moist fish, and the addition of chickpeas rounds out the meal with the needed starchy and filling high-fiber component. The beauty of keeping a well-stocked kitchen (as discussed on page 53) is that with just a few staples like chickpeas, breadcrumbs, and frozen spinach, nourishing meals are never far away. SERVES 6

6 tsp (30 mL) olive oil, divided

2 shallots, minced

1 package (10 oz/283 g) frozen spinach, thawed and squeezed to remove excess water

½ cup (125 mL) milk

Salt and pepper

2 cod filets (1 lb/450 g each)

½ cup (125 mL) Italian-style seasoned breadcrumbs, store-bought or homemade (page 244)

1 can (19 oz/540 mL) chickpeas, drained and rinsed

½ tsp (2.5 mL) crushed chili flakes

1. Preheat the oven to 350°F (180°C).

2. Heat 2 tsp (10 mL) oil in a 10-inch (25 cm) non-stick skillet set over medium heat. Add the shallots and sauté for 3 to 4 minutes, until softened. Stir in the spinach and milk, and cook for 2 minutes or until the spinach has wilted. Season with salt and pepper, remove from the heat, and let cool slightly.

3. Place one cod filet in a baking dish and season with salt and pepper. Sprinkle with half of the breadcrumbs and pat on half of the spinach mixture. Place the second cod filet on top, then the remaining spinach mixture. Top with the remaining breadcrumbs. Drizzle with 1 tsp (5 mL) olive oil.

4. In a bowl, toss the chickpeas with the remaining 3 tsp (15 mL) oil and chili flakes to coat. Arrange around the fish in the baking dish.

5. Bake for 30 minutes or until the flesh is opaque in the center and flakes easily when gently tested with a fork.

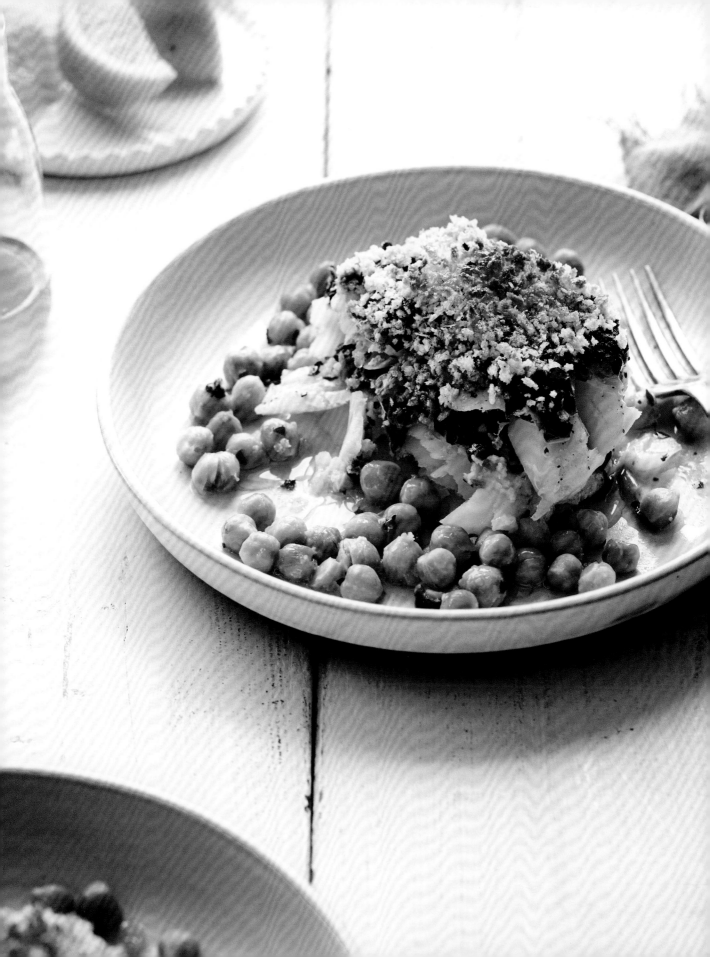

Mackerel Bucatini with Crispy Anchovy Breadcrumbs

Vegetarian • Dairy-free • Nut-free

Canned mackerel, an often overlooked ingredient, is the star of this Sicilian-inspired pasta dish. Inexpensive and high in protein and vitamin D, this oily fish is also a rich source of omega-3 fatty acids—implicated in both heart and brain health in adults, and essential for brain growth in infants. If the fishiness of mackerel has kept you away until now, this recipe is sure to win you over, with the flavorful sauce and crispy crumb topping. A simple pasta dish worthy of the best trattorias! SERVES 4 TO 6

FOR THE BREADCRUMBS

⅓ cup (80 mL) plain breadcrumbs, store-bought (such as panko) or homemade (page 244)

1 Tbsp (15 mL) olive oil

2 anchovies, finely chopped

FOR THE PASTA

2 Tbsp (30 mL) olive oil

1 onion, finely diced

2 garlic cloves, minced

1 red Italian Long Hot pepper, seeded and sliced

2 cans (4 oz/120 g each) mackerel, boneless and packed in olive oil

1 cup (250 mL) tomato purée (passata)

Salt and pepper

1 package (1 lb/450 g) bucatini

½ cup (125 mL) chopped fresh flat-leaf parsley

1. **MAKE THE BREADCRUMBS** In a small bowl, combine the breadcrumbs, oil, and anchovies. In a small, dry skillet set over medium heat, toast the anchovy breadcrumbs until golden brown, 3 minutes. Set aside in a bowl.

2. **PREPARE THE PASTA** Heat the oil in a 14-inch (35 cm) heavy-bottomed skillet set over medium heat. Add the onion and sauté for 5 minutes or until softened. Stir in the garlic and hot pepper, and cook until fragrant, 1 minute. Add the mackerel and its juice, then crumble with the back of a wooden spoon. Stir in the tomato purée, and salt and pepper to taste, then let simmer for 5 minutes.

3. Bring a large pot of salted water to a boil. Cook the pasta according to the package directions. Halfway through cooking, scoop out ½ cup (125 mL) of the pasta water and reserve. Using tongs, transfer the cooked pasta directly into the hot sauce. Add the reserved cooking water and parsley, tossing to combine. Serve and garnish with the anchovy breadcrumbs.

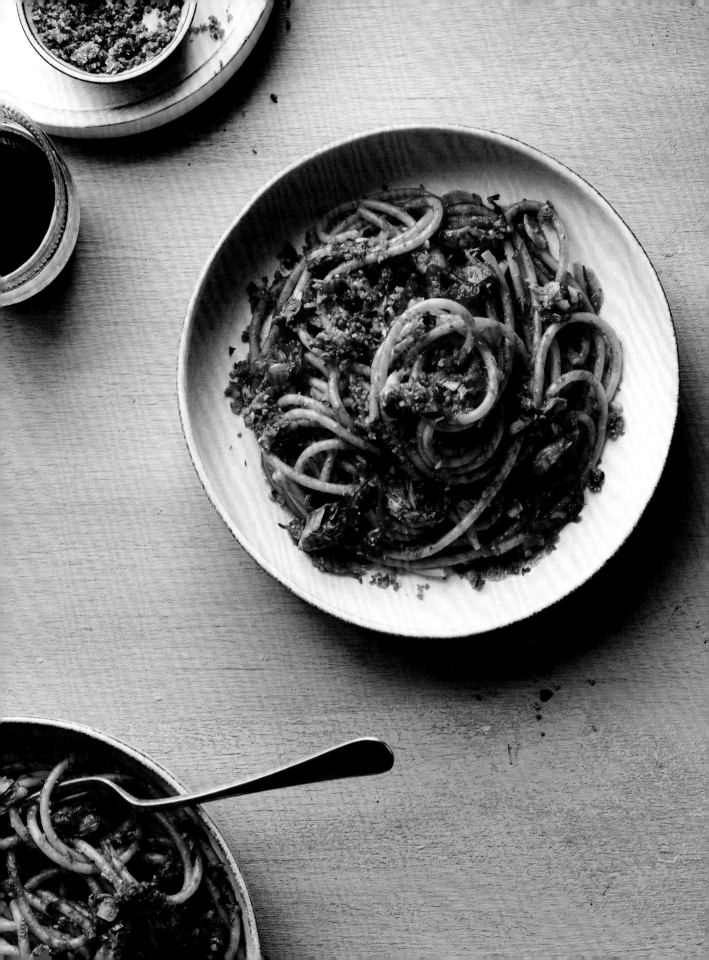

Cod in Fennel Broth

Vegetarian · Dairy-free · Gluten-free · Nut-free

My goal with this dish was to build as much flavor into the broth as quickly as possible. To achieve such a tasty result, I use clam juice—which you can find in the canned fish section at your local grocery store—and four ingredients to build up fennel flavor: fennel seeds, fennel bulb, anis liquor, and a generous handful of fresh basil. SERVES 4

2 fennel bulbs

2 Tbsp (30 mL) olive oil

½ tsp (2.5 mL) fennel seeds

¼ tsp (1 mL) crushed chili flakes

2 cups (500 mL) diced onion

3 garlic cloves, minced

½ cup (125 mL) dry white wine

3 Tbsp (45 mL) Pernod, Sambuca, or other aniseed liquor

1 can (14 oz/398 mL) diced tomatoes

1 bottle (8 oz/236 mL) clam juice

2 cups (500 mL) water

½ cup (125 mL) fresh basil

Salt and pepper

1½ lb (680 g) cod, cut into large pieces

Crusty baguette (optional)

1. Cut the fennel in half lengthwise. Using a sharp knife, make a V-shaped incision in the heart of the fennel bulb, removing the tough center while keeping the bulb intact. Remove any bruised outer layers. Thinly slice the fennel using a mandoline (set at ¼ inch/6 mm) or a knife.

2. Heat the oil in a Dutch oven set over medium heat. Add the fennel seeds and chili flakes, and cook for 30 seconds or until fragrant. Add the sliced fennel, onion, and garlic, and soften for 5 minutes, stirring frequently.

3. Deglaze with the wine and Pernod, stir, and allow to reduce for 2 minutes.

4. Add the tomatoes, clam juice, water, and basil, and season with salt and pepper. Stir to combine. Bring to a boil, reduce to a simmer, and cook the broth for 10 minutes to allow the flavors to develop.

5. Place the cod in the broth, cover, and cook at a gentle simmer for 12 minutes or until the flesh is opaque in the center and flakes easily when gently tested with a fork. Serve with a crusty baguette. Any leftovers can be stored in an airtight container in the refrigerator for up to 2 days.

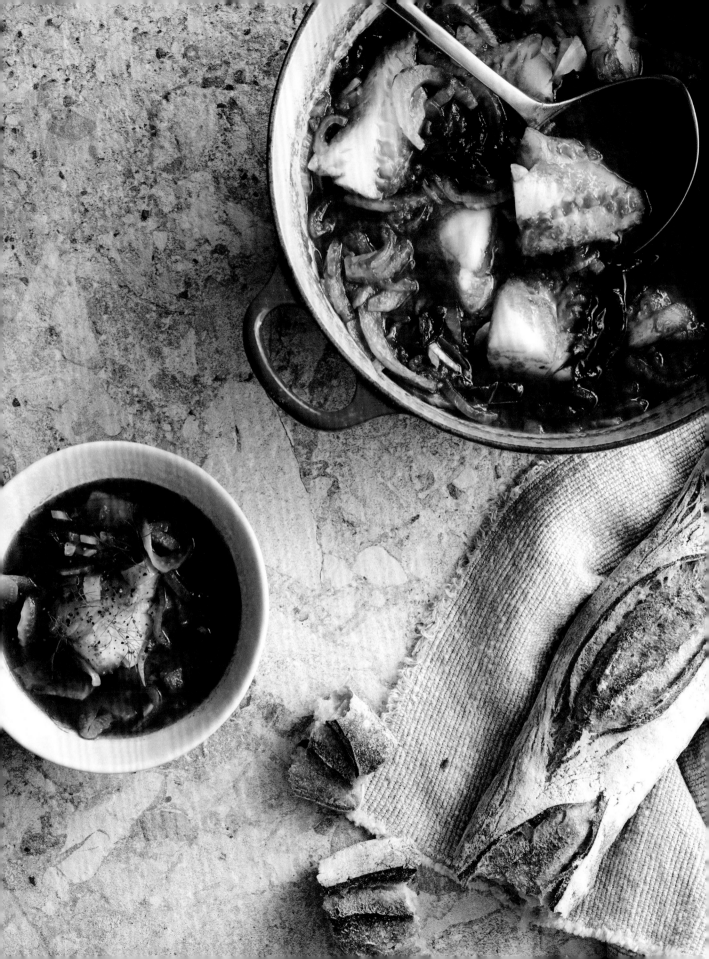

Seafood Linguine

Vegetarian • Dairy-free • Nut-free

I get it, seafood can seem intimidating if you've never prepared it before. Truth is, since we're using deveined shrimp here, this recipe comes together very quickly. In fact, by the time the pasta is done cooking, you'll have put together your sauce, so I recommend having all your ingredients prepped—this is a fast one! I like to use spelt linguine for some extra fiber in this dish and because I prefer its taste to that of whole wheat. All in all, you're in for a surprisingly simple yet elegant meal. SERVES 4 TO 6

8 oz (225 g) scallops

8 oz (225 g) shrimp (size 21/40), peeled and deveined

8 oz (225 g) squid, sliced into ½-inch-thick (1.2 cm) rings

Salt and pepper

1 package (1 lb/450 g) spelt linguine

4 Tbsp (60 mL) olive oil, divided

1 anchovy filet, minced

½ tsp (2.5 mL) crushed chili flakes

4 garlic cloves, sliced

½ cup (125 mL) dry white wine

6 Roma tomatoes, peeled, seeded, and diced (see Kitchen Tip)

½ cup (125 mL) chopped fresh flat-leaf parsley

1. Remove the muscle from each scallop by gently pulling on the tough flap on its side. Slice the scallops in half lengthwise, so they are roughly the same ½ inch (1.2 cm) thickness as the squid rings.

2. Pat all the seafood dry with paper towel. Season with salt and pepper.

3. Bring a large pot of salted water to a boil. Cook the pasta according to the package directions. Halfway through cooking, scoop out ⅓ cup (80 mL) of the pasta water and reserve.

4. Meanwhile, in a 14-inch (35 cm) skillet set over medium heat, heat 2 Tbsp (30 mL) oil. Add the anchovies and chili flakes, and cook for 30 seconds, stirring, until fragrant. Add the shrimp and garlic, and sauté for 2 minutes or until the shrimp are golden on both sides. Pour in the wine and allow it to reduce for 1 minute. Add the tomatoes, squid rings, and scallops, and cook for 3 minutes. Pour in the reserved cooking water, season with salt and pepper, cover, and cook for 3 minutes or until the seafood is opaque.

5. Using tongs, transfer the cooked pasta directly to the pan, toss, and cook for 1 minute more. Transfer the seafood linguine to a serving platter, drizzle with the remaining 2 Tbsp (30 mL) oil, garnish with the parsley, and serve. Any leftovers can be stored in an airtight container in the refrigerator for up to 2 days.

KITCHEN TIP: To peel tomatoes easily, score the bottom of each with an X, and place in a heatproof bowl. Cover with boiling water and wait 1 minute. Drain and peel.

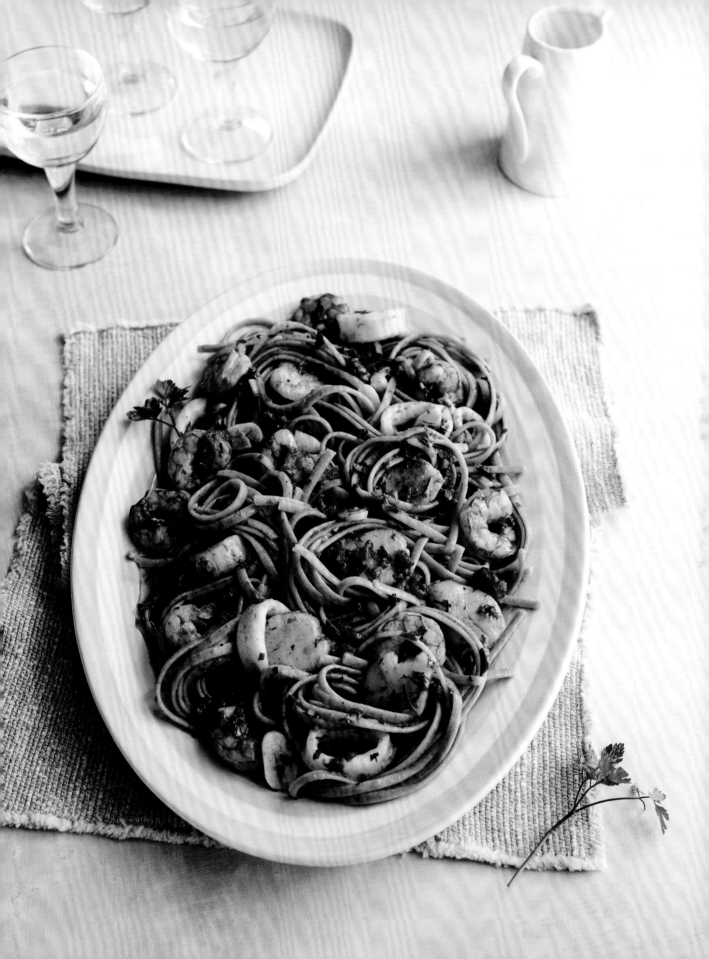

Baked Salmon with Gremolata Crust

Vegetarian • Dairy-free • Nut-free

Baked fish was the first protein I ever learned to make. It's surprisingly simple and quick, yet many still shy away from it. This recipe wraps a beautiful salmon filet in a fragrant, citrusy crust. A dish fit for a dinner party that comes together fast enough for a weeknight meal. SERVES 6

1½ lb (680 g) salmon filet

2 tsp (10 mL) Dijon mustard

1 cup (250 mL) finely chopped fresh flat-leaf parsley

½ cup (125 mL) plain breadcrumbs, store-bought (such as panko) or homemade (page 244)

1 garlic clove, minced

Zest of ½ orange

Zest of ½ lemon

1 Tbsp (15 mL) olive oil

Salt and pepper

1. Preheat the oven to 400°F (200°C) (use convection setting or for further advice, see page 61). Line a baking sheet with parchment paper.

2. Place the salmon on the prepared baking sheet and evenly brush the mustard all over.

3. In a bowl, combine the parsley, breadcrumbs, garlic, orange zest, lemon zest, oil, and a pinch each of salt and pepper. Stir to moisten the breadcrumbs evenly.

4. Cover the fish with the breadcrumb mixture, pressing firmly so it sticks to the mustard layer. Bake for 15 to 20 minutes, until the flesh is opaque in the center and flakes easily when gently tested with a fork. Serve. Any leftovers can be stored in an airtight container in the refrigerator for up to 2 days.

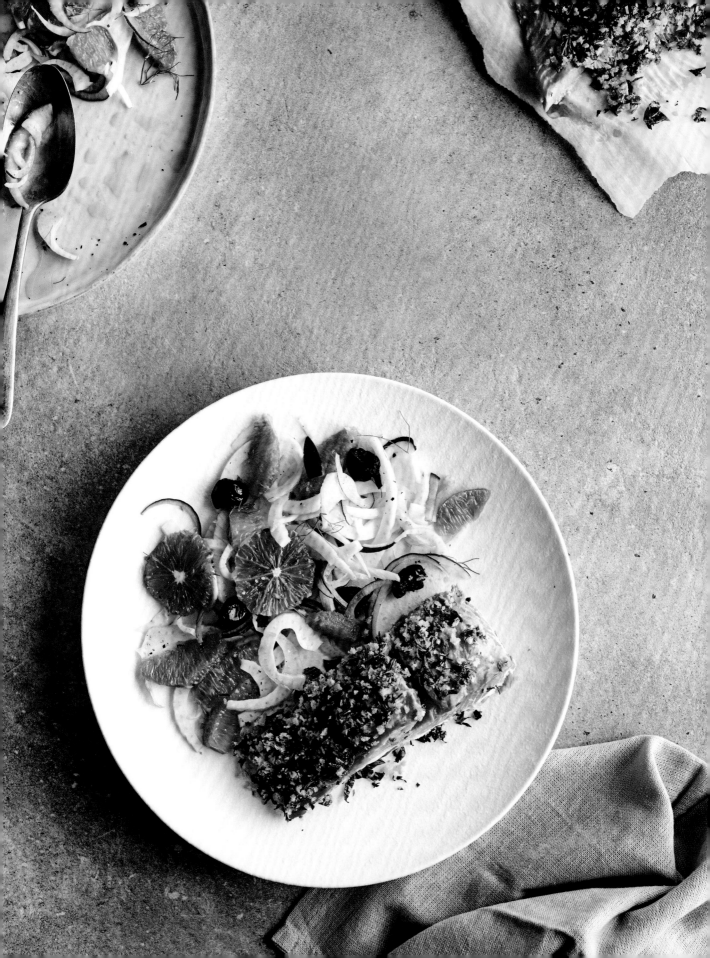

Salmon with Spanakorizo, Olives, and Tomatoes

Vegetarian • Gluten-free • Nut-free

Spanakorizo is a comforting Greek dish of spinach, rice, lemon, and dill. The rice is so packed with nutrient-dense spinach that it takes on a vibrant green color. The flavors of the spanakorizo pair wonderfully with the salmon in this recipe, making it a complete meal with the added protein. I like to use short-grain rice here because of the added creaminess it provides, resulting in a risotto-like consistency, but basmati rice can also be used, for a slightly nuttier flavor. SERVES 4

FOR THE SPANAKORIZO (SPINACH RICE)

1 Tbsp (15 mL) olive oil, plus more for drizzling

2 onions, diced

2 garlic cloves, sliced

11 oz (312 g) pre-washed baby spinach

1 cup (250 mL) short-grain white rice

3 cups (750 mL) water

Salt and pepper

¼ cup (60 mL) coarsely chopped fresh dill

¼ cup (60 mL) crumbled Greek feta

Juice of ½ lemon

FOR THE SALMON

4 salmon filets

Salt and pepper

1 cup (250 mL) halved grape tomatoes

3 Tbsp (45 mL) sliced Kalamata olives

2 Tbsp (30 mL) red wine vinegar

1. **MAKE THE SPANAKORIZO** Heat the oil in a large saucepan set over medium heat. Add the onion and garlic, and cook for 5 minutes or until softened. Add the spinach and stir constantly until wilted, 2 minutes. Add the rice, water, and salt and pepper to taste and bring to a boil. Cover, reduce the heat to medium-low, and cook for 20 minutes without stirring. Stir in the dill and feta, then remove from the heat. Drizzle with the lemon juice and another drizzle of olive oil, if desired. Set aside and keep warm.

2. Preheat the oven to 400°F (200°C). Line a baking sheet with parchment paper.

3. **PREPARE THE SALMON** Place the salmon on the prepared baking sheet. Season with salt and pepper. Bake for 15 to 18 minutes, until the flesh is opaque in the center and flakes easily when gently tested with a fork.

4. In a small bowl, combine the tomatoes, olives, and vinegar. Serve the salmon, garnished with the tomato mixture, with the rice on the side. Any leftovers can be stored in an airtight container in the refrigerator for up to 2 days.

Broiled Halibut with Pistachio Pesto and Asparagus

Vegetarian • Dairy-free • Gluten-free

I love a good sheet-pan dinner. In this case, the broiler makes it come together very quickly. The fish, cooked on a bed of lemon, is smothered in an herby pistachio pesto that creates a flavorful crust loaded with healthy fat and fiber. It's a weeknight staple worthy of company, and a dish in which any firm white fish would shine. SERVES 4

1. **MAKE THE PESTO** In a food processor fitted with a steel blade, pulse the basil, mint, pistachios, garlic, salt to taste, and chili flakes until finely chopped. With the motor still running, slowly pour in the oil, blending until smooth. Adjust the seasoning to taste. Divide the pesto between two bowls.

2. Preheat the broiler to high and set the oven rack 6 inches (15 cm) from the element. Line a baking sheet with aluminum foil.

3. **MAKE THE HALIBUT** Lay the lemon slices in four rows on the prepared baking sheet. This will serve as a bed for each filet.

4. Season the fish on both sides with salt and pepper. Place each filet on a lemon row and brush with some of the reserved pesto (each time from the same bowl so as not to cross-contaminate). Arrange the asparagus around the fish. Drizzle with the oil, then gently toss the asparagus using your hands. Season with salt and pepper.

5. Broil for 10 to 12 minutes, until the flesh is opaque in the center and flakes easily when gently tested with a fork. Serve with a dollop of the reserved pesto (from the second bowl). Any leftover fish can be stored in an airtight container in the refrigerator for up to 2 days. Any leftover pesto can be stored in an airtight container in the refrigerator for up to 4 days or in the freezer for up to 6 months.

FOR THE PESTO

2 cups (500 mL) fresh basil

½ cup (125 mL) fresh mint

½ cup (125 mL) unsalted pistachios

2 cloves garlic

Pinch of salt

⅛ tsp (0.5 mL) crushed chili flakes

½ cup (125 mL) extra virgin olive oil

FOR THE HALIBUT

2 lemons, cut into ¼-inch-thick (6 mm) rounds

4 Pacific halibut (or other firm white fish) filets (6 oz/170 g each)

Kosher salt

Freshly cracked black pepper

1 bunch of asparagus, ends trimmed

1 Tbsp (15 mL) olive oil

Shrimp and Tomato Skewers

Vegetarian • Dairy-free • Gluten-free • Nut-free

I keep frozen shrimp on hand, since they are a quick-cooking and versatile way to add protein to a meal. In this recipe, the paprika and herb marinade adds smokiness to the shrimp, complemented by bursts of sweet, juicy tomatoes. I like to make a double batch of this flavorful marinade and freeze extras in an ice cube tray, so I'm prepared for a no-fuss weeknight recipe or an impromptu appetizer. Outside of grilling season, a cast-iron grill pan set over high heat will also do the trick. SERVES 4

2 lb (1 kg) shrimp (size 21/40), peeled, deveined

2 cups (500 mL) cherry tomatoes

¼ cup (60 mL) olive oil

½ cup (125 mL) fresh flat-leaf parsley

¼ cup (60 mL) fresh basil

2 Tbsp (30 mL) fresh oregano

1 tsp (5 mL) paprika

½ tsp (2.5 mL) crushed chili flakes

Zest and juice of 1 lemon

4 garlic cloves

Salt and pepper

1. Place the shrimp and tomatoes in a bowl.

2. In a food processor fitted with a steel blade, process the oil, parsley, basil, oregano, paprika, chili flakes, lemon zest, lemon juice, and garlic until smooth. Pour over the shrimp and tomatoes, tossing to coat. Cover and marinate in the refrigerator for 30 minutes.

3. Preheat the barbecue to high and oil the grates. If using wooden skewers, soak eight 10- to 12-inch (25 to 30 cm) skewers in water for at least 5 minutes.

4. Thread the shrimp and tomatoes, alternating, onto skewers and season with salt and pepper to taste. Discard the marinade. Grill the skewers for 2 to 4 minutes on each side, until the shrimp are well browned and opaque. Enjoy right away.

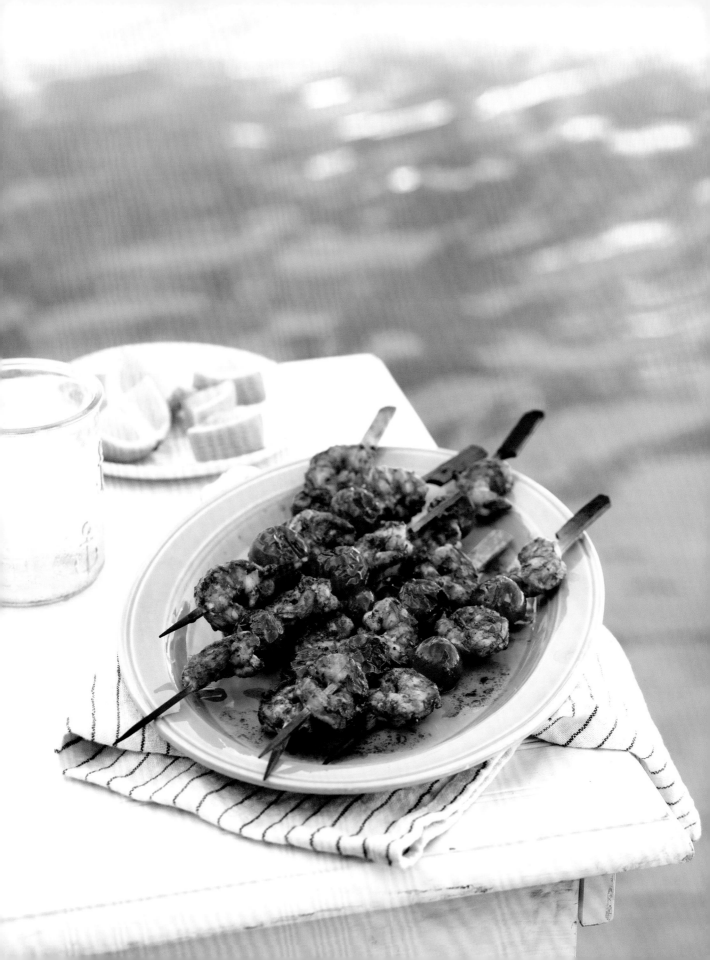

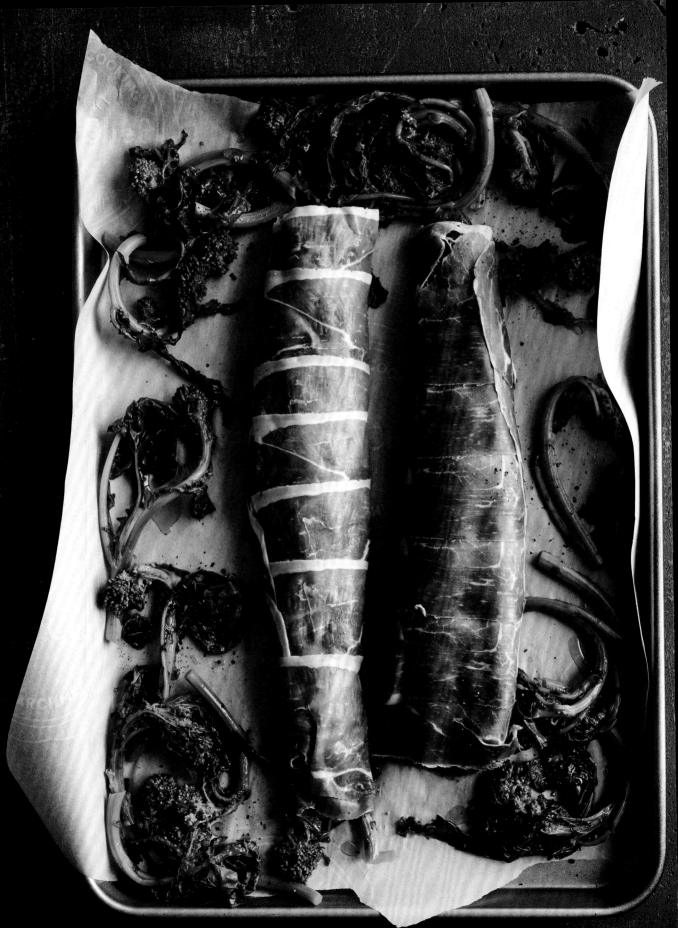

Meat

Modest means and a lack of accessibility made cooking and eating meat a rare occurrence for those observing the traditional Mediterranean diet. And despite better access to these foods today, there is still reason to moderate our meat consumption, be it nutritional or environmental. Keeping with the principles of the Mediterranean diet, poultry dishes are eaten a couple of times per week—Greek Chicken Burgers (page 206) and Balsamic Braised Chicken with Onions and Olives (page 198) are two of my go-to weeknight meals. Red meat, on the other hand, appears less frequently, on a weekly or bi-weekly basis—try the delicious Flank Steak Salad with Crispy White Beans (page 204). One thing is for certain: when meat is on the menu, it is to be savored and celebrated.

Nonna's Veal Stew

Dairy-free • Nut-free

To me, there is almost nothing more comforting than a bowl of homemade stew. Perhaps it's because the dish takes me back to my grandmother's kitchen, as most memorable meals also do. This was one of her go-to recipes, since stewing allowed her to build flavor and tenderize tougher, more affordable cuts of meat. All cuts of meat are more costly today than they once were, but the fact that this recipe comes together in one pot, is a complete meal, and is freezer-friendly and therefore batch-cooking-friendly, makes it worth it in my book. SERVES 6

2 lb (1 kg) boneless veal shoulder, cubed

2 Tbsp (30 mL) all-purpose flour

Salt and pepper

2 Tbsp (30 mL) olive oil, divided

2 onions, diced

2 celery stalks, sliced

2 garlic cloves, minced

½ cup (125 mL) dry white wine

2 cups (500 mL) low-sodium beef broth

4 red potatoes, peeled and quartered

1 bay leaf

1 cup (250 mL) frozen green peas

½ cup (125 mL) chopped fresh flat-leaf parsley

1. In a bowl, toss the veal with the flour and salt and pepper to taste, ensuring it's evenly coated.

2. Heat 1 Tbsp (15 mL) oil in a large pot set over medium-high heat. Add the veal and brown on all sides, 7 to 8 minutes. Transfer to a plate.

3. Reduce the heat to medium, add the remaining 1 Tbsp (15 mL) oil, along with the onion, celery, and garlic, and sauté for 5 minutes or until the vegetables have softened. Deglaze with the wine and allow to reduce, 2 minutes.

4. Return the veal to the pot and add the broth, potatoes, bay leaf, and a pinch of salt and pepper. Bring to a boil, reduce to a simmer, cover, and cook for 40 minutes or until the meat is fork-tender.

5. Adjust the seasoning to taste, add the peas, and continue to simmer for 5 more minutes or until the peas are cooked and bright green. Garnish with the parsley and serve. Any leftovers can be stored in an airtight container in the refrigerator for up to 4 days or in the freezer for up to 3 months.

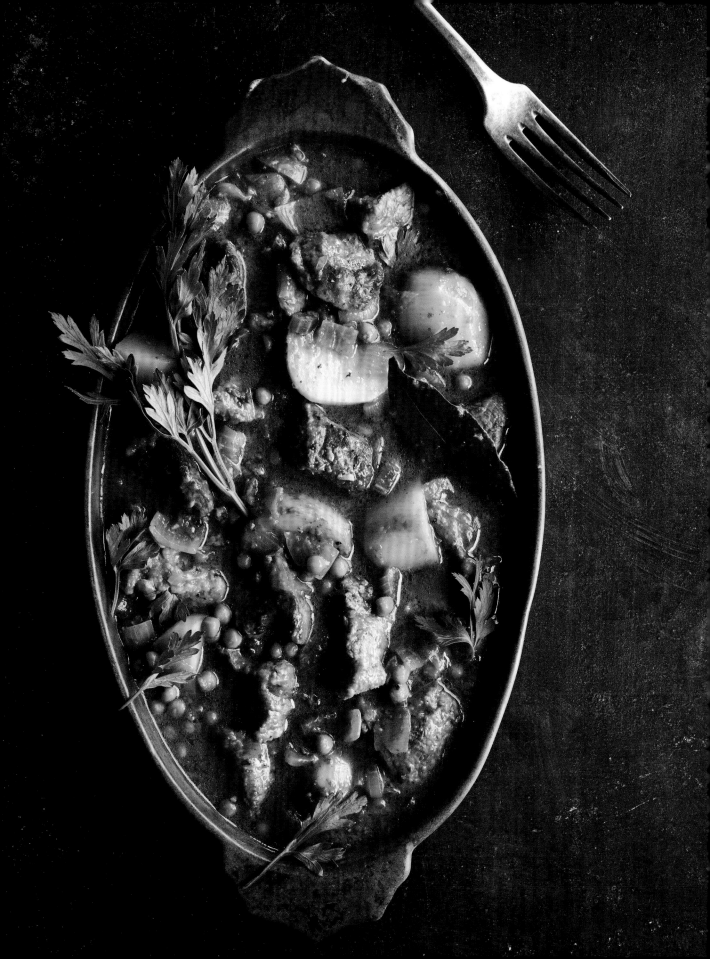

Pork Souvlaki Pitas

Nut-free

I love a good homemade rendition of a restaurant classic, and these Greek pitas certainly fit the bill. The marinade combines citrusy coriander seeds with earthy oregano and thyme, spices that are chock-full of beneficial compounds as well as flavor. Topped with sharp tzatziki and your favorite pita fixings, this dish will give you all the satisfaction you'd expect and more. The soft Greek Yogurt Flatbreads (page 109) are my preferred choice for this recipe, but if you're short on time, any soft store-bought pita will do. SERVES 6

FOR THE PORK

¼ cup (60 mL) olive oil

2 Tbsp (30 mL) red wine vinegar

Zest and juice of 1 lemon

4 garlic cloves, minced

2 tsp (10 mL) coriander seeds, crushed

1 Tbsp (15 mL) dried oregano

1 tsp (5 mL) dried thyme

2 pork tenderloins (about 1 lb/450 g each), cut into 1-inch (2.5 cm) pieces (see Kitchen Tip)

Salt and pepper

TO ASSEMBLE

6 pitas or flatbreads, store-bought or homemade (page 109)

Tzatziki sauce, store-bought or homemade (page 249)

2 tomatoes, sliced

1 red onion, thinly sliced

6 romaine lettuce leaves, shredded

1. In a large bowl, whisk together the oil, vinegar, lemon zest, lemon juice, garlic, coriander seeds, oregano, and thyme. Add the pork, mixing well to coat the meat. Cover and marinate in the refrigerator for at least 1 hour and up to overnight.

2. Heat a barbecue or grill pan to medium-high. If using wooden skewers, soak eight 10- to 12-inch (25 to 30 cm) skewers in water for at least 5 minutes.

3. Season the pork with salt and pepper to taste. Thread the pork cubes onto the skewers.

4. Grill the skewers for about 12 to 15 minutes, turning every 3 minutes until all sides of the pork are browned and the meat is cooked through (with an internal temperature of 160°F/71°C).

5. Serve each skewer alongside a pita bread and garnish with tzatziki, tomatoes, onion, and lettuce. Any leftover souvlaki can be stored in an airtight container in the refrigerator for up to 3 days.

KITCHEN TIP: You can replace the pork with the same amount of boneless, skinless chicken breast, if desired.

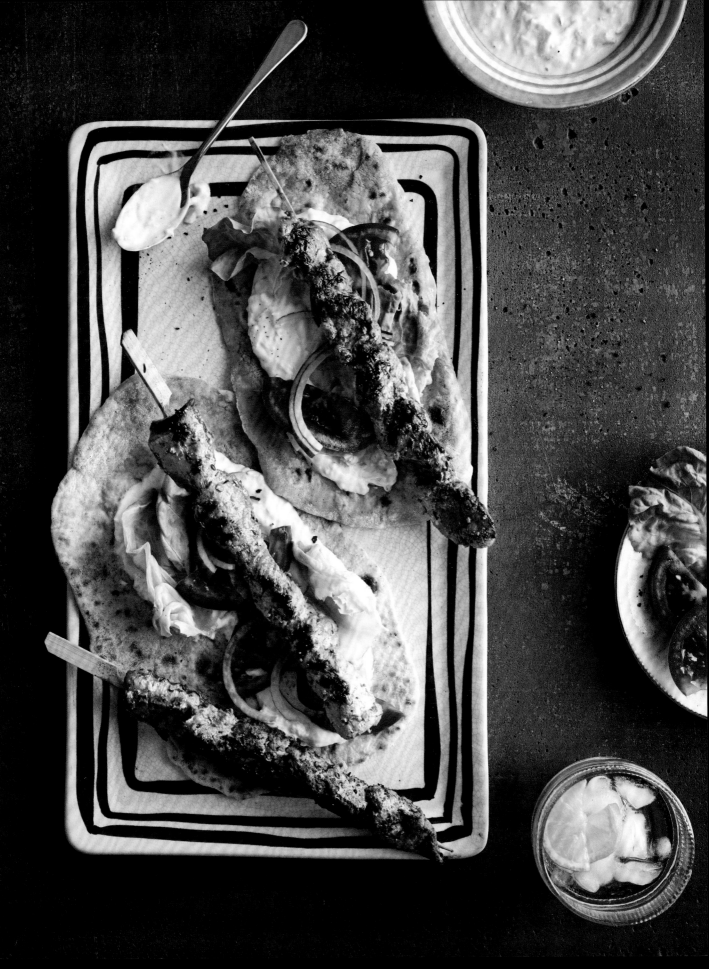

Spiced Chicken Drumsticks with Parsnip Fries

Gluten-free • Nut-free

Harissa is a spicy Tunisian pepper paste made from peppers, garlic, and spices like paprika, coriander, and caraway. It packs heat and makes a flavorful marinade for these drumsticks. Parsnip is a sweet-tasting root vegetable and chock-full of vitamin C; it makes for the perfect fries for this spicy main. SERVES 4 TO 6

FOR THE DRUMSTICKS

¼ cup (60 mL) plain yogurt

3 Tbsp (45 mL) olive oil

2 Tbsp (30 mL) harissa paste (see Kitchen Tip)

1 tsp (5 mL) smoked paprika

1 tsp (5 mL) ground cumin

1 tsp (5 mL) ground coriander

6 garlic cloves, minced

Salt and pepper

10 chicken drumsticks (about 2 lb/1 kg)

FOR THE PARSNIP FRIES

1 lb (454 g) parsnips, peeled and cut into sticks about ¼ inch (6 mm) thick and 4 inches (10 cm) long

1 Tbsp (15 mL) olive oil

½ tsp (2.5 mL) sumac

Salt and pepper

1. **PREPARE THE DRUMSTICKS** In a large bowl, whisk together the yogurt, oil, harissa, paprika, cumin, coriander, garlic, and salt and pepper to taste. Add the chicken and toss to evenly coat. Cover and marinate in the refrigerator for at least 4 hours and up to overnight.

2. Preheat the oven to 425°F (220°C). Line a baking sheet with aluminum foil and lightly oil.

3. Remove the chicken from the refrigerator as the oven preheats to bring to room temperature. Season with salt and pepper, and place on the prepared baking sheet. Bake drumsticks 45 to 50 minutes, stirring frequently, until nicely browned and cooked through.

4. **PREPARE THE PARSNIP FRIES** Meanwhile, line another baking sheet with parchment paper. Place the parsnips on the prepared baking sheet and drizzle with the oil. Sprinkle the sumac overtop, and season with salt and pepper. Toss and spread out evenly on the baking sheet. Roast in the oven at the end of the chicken's cooking time, for 20 to 25 minutes, until golden brown. Adjust the seasoning to taste, and serve with the chicken. Any leftovers can be stored in an airtight container in the refrigerator for up to 3 days.

KITCHEN TIP: Harissa paste, sold in a tube, can be found in the condiments aisle of the grocery store.

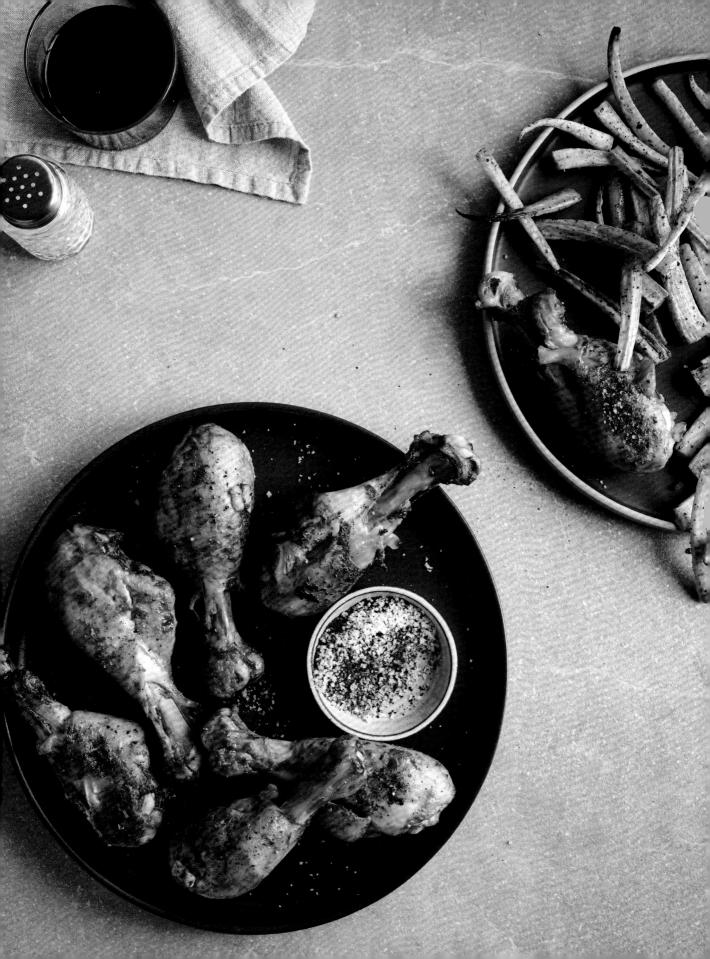

Za'atar Grilled Chicken Salad

Dairy-free · Gluten-free · Nut-free

In this recipe, za'atar packs the chicken with flavor, and a hot grill pan is the secret to locking in its moisture. The juicy chicken is then placed on a big bowl of crisp romaine, fresh vegetables, and creamy avocado topped with a zippy dressing. This salad exceeds the three-color-per-plate goal for powering up (page 29), and also exceeds flavor expectations. Makes for a great workday lunch or lighter dinner. SERVES 4

FOR THE CHICKEN

2 boneless, skinless chicken breasts (about 1 lb/450g)

1 Tbsp (15 mL) extra virgin olive oil

3 Tbsp (45 mL) za'atar

½ tsp (2.5 mL) garlic powder

Salt and pepper

FOR THE DRESSING

¼ cup (60 mL) extra virgin olive oil

Juice of 1 lemon

1 garlic clove, minced

2 Tbsp (30 mL) chopped parsley

2 tsp (10 mL) dried mint

Salt and pepper

FOR THE SALAD

4 cups (1 L) romaine lettuce, chopped

4 radishes, sliced

2 Roma tomatoes, diced

2 Persian cucumbers, sliced

1 avocado, pitted, peeled, and sliced

¼ red onion, thinly sliced

1. **PREPARE THE CHICKEN** Slice each chicken breast in half horizontally. Place the chicken in a bowl and add the oil, za'atar, garlic powder, and salt and pepper to taste. Toss to coat, cover, and let marinate in the refrigerator for 30 minutes.

2. Heat a grill pan or cast-iron skillet over medium-high heat. Grill the chicken for 12 to 15 minutes, turning halfway through, until the internal temperature reaches 165°F (74°C). Transfer to a cutting board and let rest for 2 minutes before slicing into strips.

3. **MAKE THE DRESSING** In a small bowl, whisk together the oil, lemon juice, garlic, parsley, mint, and salt and pepper to taste.

4. **MAKE THE SALAD AND SERVE** In a large bowl, toss the lettuce, radishes, tomatoes, cucumbers, avocado, and onion with the dressing. Divide among individual bowls and top with the chicken. Any leftovers can be stored in an airtight container in the refrigerator for up to 3 days.

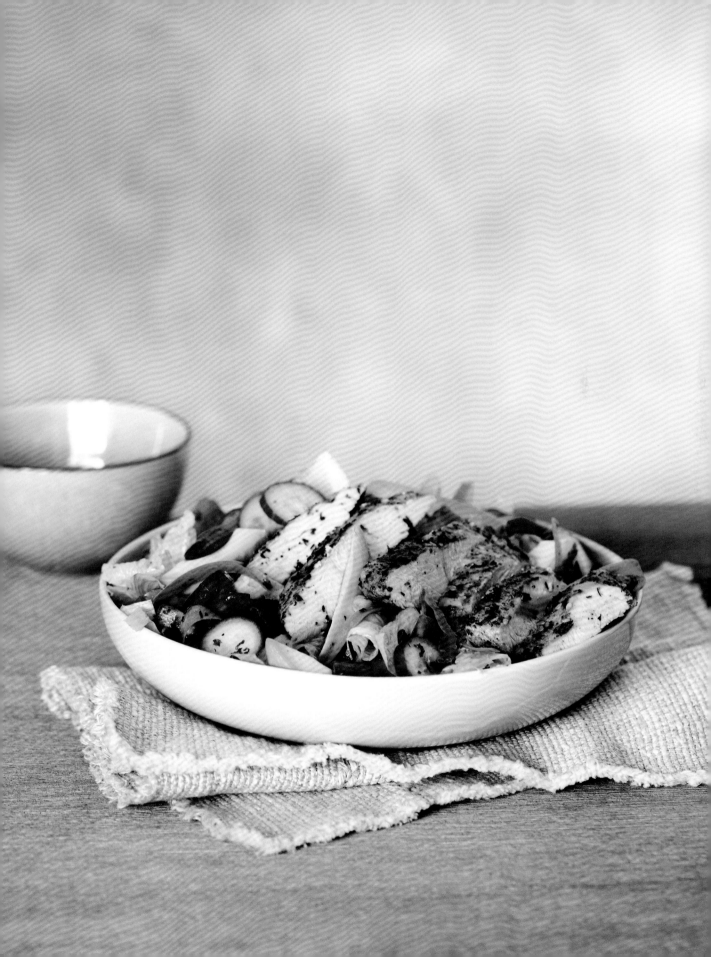

Balsamic Braised Chicken with Onions and Olives

Dairy-free • Gluten-free • Nut-free

Don't let the simple ingredients list fool you; this one-pot recipe delivers big on flavor. Tender chicken, jammy onions, and briny olives take on sweet and sour notes thanks to a duo of balsamic vinegar and honey, and come together similar to a chicken cacciatore, but *better*. I love to serve this saucy dish with rice and pair it with the Everyday Green Salad (page 136) for an extra helping of vegetables. SERVES 6

12 boneless, skinless chicken thighs (about 2 lb/1 kg)

Salt and pepper

3 Tbsp (45 mL) olive oil, divided

3 cups (750 mL) chopped onion

3 garlic cloves, minced

2 anchovies, chopped, or 1 tsp (5 mL) anchovy paste

½ cup (125 mL) aged balsamic vinegar (see Kitchen Tip)

1 Tbsp (15 mL) honey

1 cup (250 mL) tomato purée (passata)

1 cup (250 mL) pitted green olives

3 sprigs of thyme

1 bay leaf

2 Tbsp (30 mL) chopped parsley

2 cups (500 mL) cooked brown rice, to serve (optional)

1. Season the chicken with salt and pepper to taste on both sides.

2. Heat 1 Tbsp (15 mL) oil in a large Dutch oven set over medium-high heat. Working in batches, brown the chicken thighs for 2 to 3 minutes per side. Set aside on a plate.

3. Reduce the heat to medium and add the remaining 2 Tbsp (30 mL) oil, along with the onion, garlic, and anchovies. Sauté for 5 minutes or until softened.

4. Stir in the vinegar and honey, and reduce by half, about 2 minutes.

5. Add the tomato purée, olives, thyme, bay leaf, and chicken. Stir to coat the chicken in the sauce. Season with salt and pepper, bring to a simmer, cover, and cook for 20 minutes. Adjust the seasoning to taste and simmer, uncovered, for 5 minutes more or until the chicken is cooked through. Garnish with parsley and serve with rice or your favorite whole grain. Any leftovers can be stored in an airtight container in the refrigerator for up to 3 days or in the freezer for up to 3 months.

KITCHEN TIP: Balsamic vinegar has a complex, sweet taste. It can be used in vinaigrettes, in desserts, or when cooking, as in this recipe, to deglaze a pan. Traditional balsamic vinegar bears the label "DOP"—standing for "Denominazione di Origine Protetta"—a guarantee of quality and authenticity.

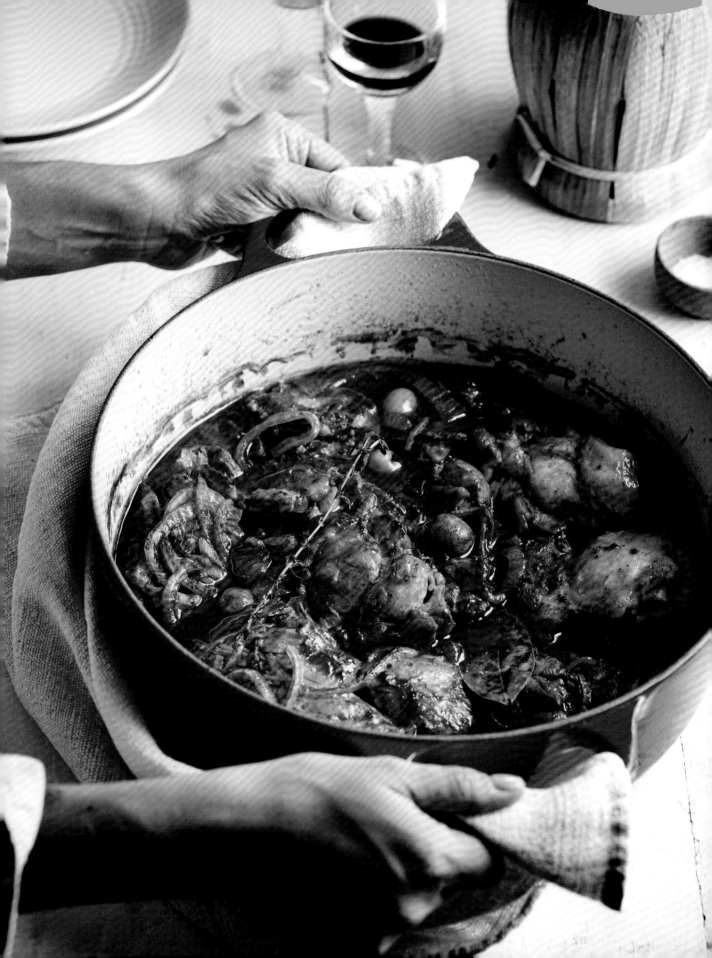

Porchetta-Style Tenderloin with Rapini

Dairy-free • Gluten-free • Nut-free

When my father prepares his annual porchetta, the whole family reunites for the occasion. This recipe is inspired by the flavors of this yearly tradition, but simplified to fit an everyday meal. Traditional woodsy herbs and spices such as sage, fennel seeds, and chili, along with garlic, flavor the center of the pork tenderloin, which is wrapped in thin slices of prosciutto to impart flavor, mimicking the traditional pork belly in a porchetta roll. I always recommend being liberal with herbs and spices in meat dishes not only because of their flavor-enhancing characteristics but also because their natural antioxidants may offer protection against harmful compounds produced in heated meat. I love thinly slicing any leftovers and adding to a ciabatta with salsa verde, for a delicious sandwich the next day. SERVES 6

1 Tbsp (15 mL) fennel seeds

4 sage leaves, sliced

3 garlic cloves, minced

½ cup (125 mL) coarsely chopped fresh flat-leaf parsley

2 Tbsp (30 mL) fresh rosemary (about 1 sprig)

½ tsp (2.5 mL) crushed chili flakes

½ tsp (2.5 mL) freshly cracked black pepper

2 Tbsp (30 mL) olive oil

2 pork tenderloins (1 lb/450 g each)

Salt and pepper

10 slices of prosciutto

1 bunch of rapini (broccoli rabe), ends trimmed

Salsa Verde (page 250), to serve (optional)

1. Preheat the oven to 400°F (200°C). Line a baking sheet with parchment paper.

2. In a small, dry skillet set over medium heat, toast the fennel seeds, stirring occasionally, until fragrant, about 2 minutes.

3. In a mortar and pestle (or a food processor), grind the toasted fennel seeds, sage, garlic, parsley, rosemary, chili flakes, pepper, and oil to a paste.

4. Butterfly each pork tenderloin by slicing them horizontally and stopping midway, so that they open like books. Spread the meat and pound it to a ½ inch (1.2 cm) even thickness. Season the meat with salt and pepper to taste and brush with the herb paste. Roll the filets firmly lengthwise, then wrap each log with five slices of prosciutto. Place the tenderloins in the center of the prepared baking sheet.

5. Bring a large pot of water to a boil. Cook the rapini for 1 minute, then drain well. Lay the rapini around the pork, drizzle the greens with olive oil, and season with salt and pepper. Roast for 25 to 30 minutes or until the internal temperature reaches 160°F (71°C). Tent the pork with foil and let rest for 5 minutes before slicing. Serve with the salsa verde. Any leftover pork can be stored in an airtight container in the refrigerator for up to 3 days.

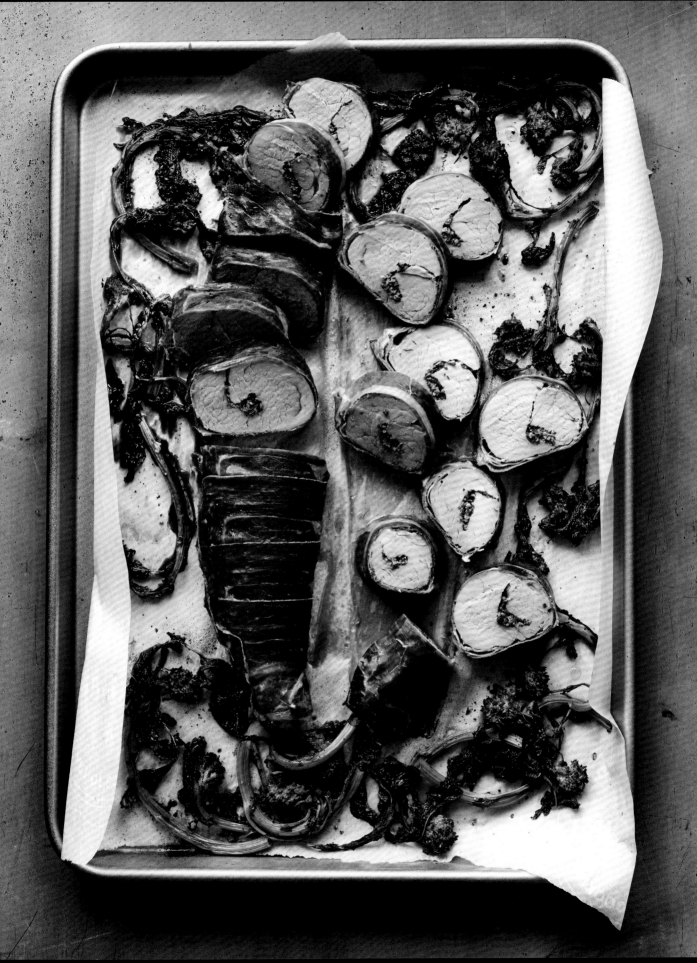

Kefta Kebabs and Mast-o Khiar

Gluten-free

Mast-o khiar is a delicious and cooling Persian yogurt and cucumber salad, and the perfect pairing for these spiced skewers. Cumin, paprika, coriander, and cayenne flavor these half-beef, half-lamb kebabs that are great for a weeknight meal or fit for a barbecue with friends. I like to serve these with the Kale Fattoush (page 102) for greens and color. For the lamb-averse, these can be prepared using all beef. SERVES 6

FOR THE KEBABS

1 lb (450 g) extra-lean ground beef

1 lb (450 g) ground lamb

4 garlic cloves, minced

1 onion, grated

2 Tbsp (30 mL) tomato paste

1 Tbsp (15 mL) ground coriander

2 tsp (10 mL) ground cumin

1 tsp (5 mL) paprika

½ tsp (2.5 mL) cayenne pepper

Salt and pepper

FOR THE MAST-O KHIAR

1 cup (250 mL) plain Greek yogurt

2 Persian cucumbers, grated and pressed of excess water

1 garlic clove, minced

¼ cup (60 mL) chopped fresh mint

1 Tbsp (15 mL) raisins

1 Tbsp (15 mL) chopped toasted walnuts

Salt and pepper

1. **PREPARE THE KEFTA KEBABS** Heat the barbecue to medium-high and oil the grates. If using wooden skewers, soak twelve 10- to 12-inch (25 to 30 cm) wooden skewers in water at least 5 minutes.

2. In a large bowl and using your hands, mix together the beef, lamb, garlic, onion, tomato paste, coriander, cumin, paprika, cayenne, and salt and pepper to taste. Divide the mixture into 12 portions and shape into long meatballs directly on the pre-soaked skewers. Leave 1 to 2 inches (2.5 to 5 cm) at one end of the skewer empty, to make for easier handling. Set aside on a plate.

3. Grill the kefta kebabs with the lid of the barbecue closed, about 6 minutes per side, until nicely browned and cooked through.

4. **PREPARE THE MAST-O KHIAR** In a small bowl, combine the yogurt, cucumbers, garlic, mint, raisins, and walnuts. Season with salt and pepper, and serve with the kefta kebabs. Any leftovers can be stored in an airtight container in the refrigerator for up to 3 days.

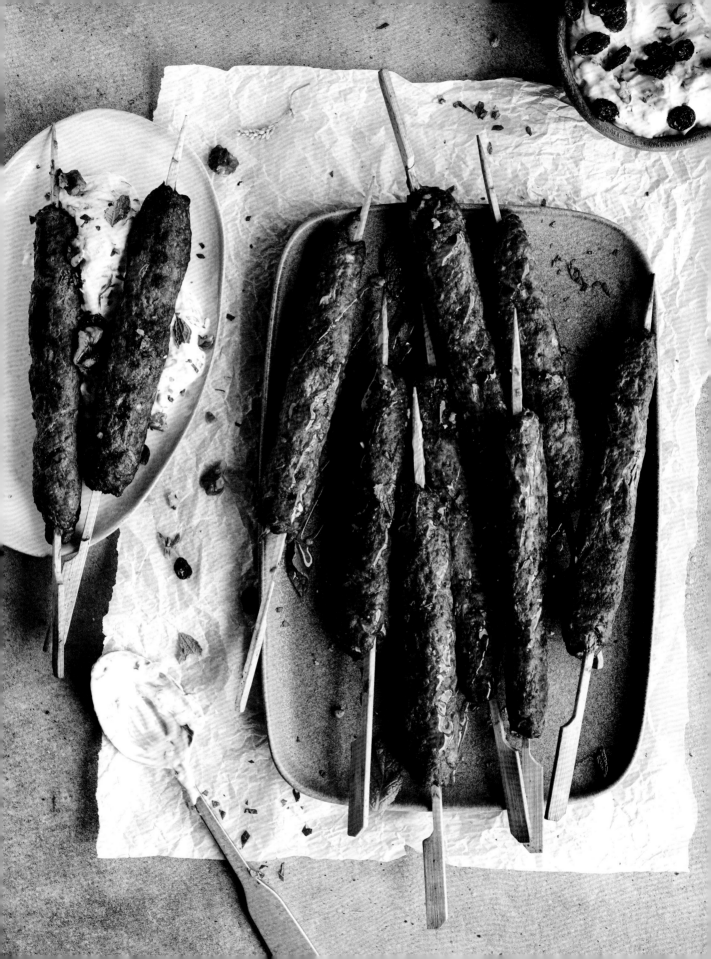

Flank Steak Salad with Crispy White Beans

Dairy-free · Gluten-free · Nut-free

Red meat isn't a prominent part of the Mediterranean diet, so for those people used to eating it regularly, using plant-based proteins like beans in meals can help reduce meat portions. This is a great example of a positive, "eat more" strategy, one that focuses on *adding* something nutritious to the diet, in contrast to the unsustainable "avoid" rhetoric we are often sold by diet culture. The fact is, plant-based proteins like beans are a delicious stepping stone for those carnivores aspiring to plant-power their diets! In this dish, white beans are crisped up in the oven, acting like protein-packed croutons on top of this peppery salad. They also make for a great crunchy snack. SERVES 4 TO 6

FOR THE STEAK

1 lb (450 g) flank steak

2 Tbsp (30 mL) olive oil

2 Tbsp (30 mL) balsamic vinegar

2 garlic cloves, crushed

1 sprig of rosemary, leaves stripped

Salt and pepper

FOR THE SALAD

1 can (19 oz/540 mL) white kidney or cannellini beans, drained and rinsed

4 garlic cloves, crushed

1 sprig of rosemary, leaves stripped

1 Tbsp (15 mL) olive oil

Salt and pepper

4 cups (1 L) packed arugula

2 cups (500 mL) halved cherry tomatoes

Salsa Verde (page 250)

1. **PREPARE THE STEAK** Score the steak lightly to allow some of the marinade to permeate the meat. Place the meat in a resealable bag with the oil, vinegar, garlic, rosemary, and salt and pepper to taste. Seal the bag, massage the meat with the other ingredients, and then refrigerate for at least 30 minutes and up to overnight.

2. Preheat the oven to 425°F (220°C). Line a baking sheet with parchment paper.

3. **PREPARE THE SALAD** Pat the beans dry with a clean kitchen towel. Transfer to a bowl with the garlic, rosemary, oil, and salt and pepper to taste. Toss, then spread evenly on the prepared baking sheet. Roast for 30 minutes, stirring halfway through, until the beans are golden brown.

4. Heat a large cast-iron skillet over medium-high heat. Remove the steak from the marinade, discarding the marinade. Sear the steak in the hot pan for 6 minutes per side for medium doneness, or until desired doneness. Transfer to a cutting board, tent with aluminum foil, and let rest for 10 minutes. Slice the meat against the grain and transfer to a serving platter.

5. Arrange the arugula around the meat, and top both with the roasted beans and tomatoes. Drizzle with the salsa verde and serve. Any leftover steak can be stored in an airtight container in the refrigerator for up to 3 days.

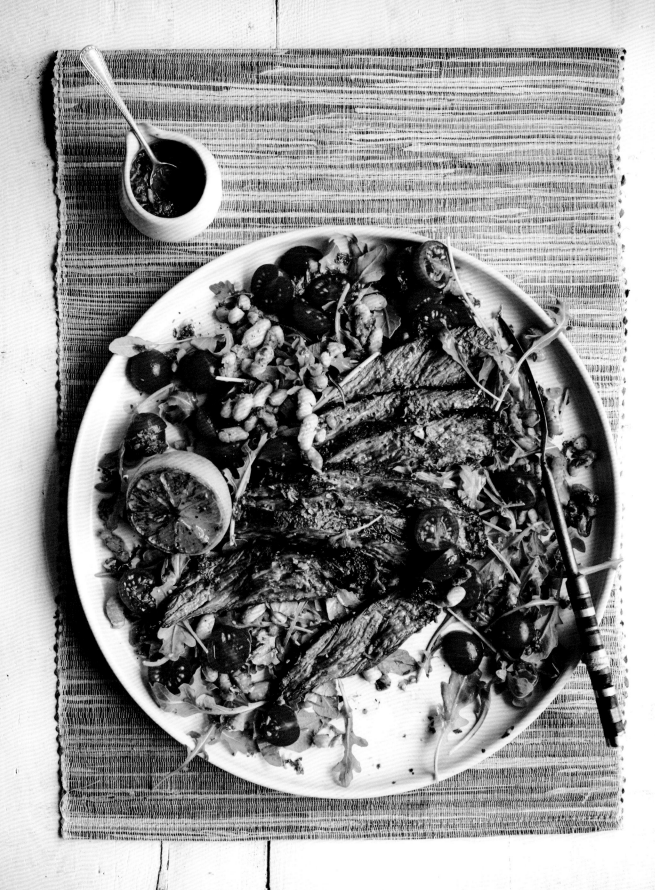

Greek Chicken Burgers

Nut-free

These burgers are like a deconstructed Greek salad in a bun. Flavorful patties with specks of spinach and sun-dried tomatoes are topped with a feta yogurt spread, crisp cucumber, tangy tomato, and sharp red onion. Although these burgers contain vegetables in every layer, serve alongside the Everyday Green Salad (page 136) for an extra helping of greens and fiber. MAKES 6 BURGERS

FOR THE PATTIES

1 tsp (5 mL) olive oil

1 red onion, finely diced

1 garlic clove, minced

½ cup (125 mL) frozen chopped spinach, thawed and pressed of excess water

½ cup (125 mL) sun-dried tomatoes, finely chopped

1½ lb (680 g) ground chicken

1 egg, lightly beaten

Salt and pepper

FOR THE FETA YOGURT SPREAD

½ cup (125 mL) full-fat Greek yogurt

½ cup (125 mL) crumbled feta

2 Tbsp (30 mL) coarsely chopped fresh dill

Juice of ½ lemon

TO ASSEMBLE

6 burger buns

2 Persian cucumbers, cut into strips

2 tomatoes, sliced

6 leaves of butter lettuce

½ red onion, sliced

1. **PREPARE THE PATTIES** Heat the oil in a 10-inch (25 cm) non-stick skillet set over medium-high heat. Add the onion, garlic, and spinach, and sauté for 5 minutes or until the onion is softened.

2. Stir in the sun-dried tomatoes, then remove from the heat and let cool slightly.

3. Place the ground chicken in a large bowl along with the egg and spinach mixture and season with salt and pepper. Mix well, using your hands, and divide into six patties. Refrigerate the patties, covered on a plate, until ready to use.

4. **PREPARE THE SPREAD** Blend the yogurt, cheese, dill, and lemon juice in a blender until smooth.

5. Heat a barbecue or a grill pan to medium-high and oil the grates. Grill the patties until golden and cooked through, about 6 to 8 minutes per side. Meanwhile, toast the buns.

6. **ASSEMBLE THE BURGERS** Place a generous dollop of the spread on the bun bottoms, then top with the patties, cucumbers, tomatoes, lettuce, onion, and bun tops. Any leftover patties can be stored in an airtight container in the refrigerator for up to 3 days or in the freezer for up to 3 months. Any leftover feta spread can be stored in an airtight container in the refrigerator for up to 3 days.

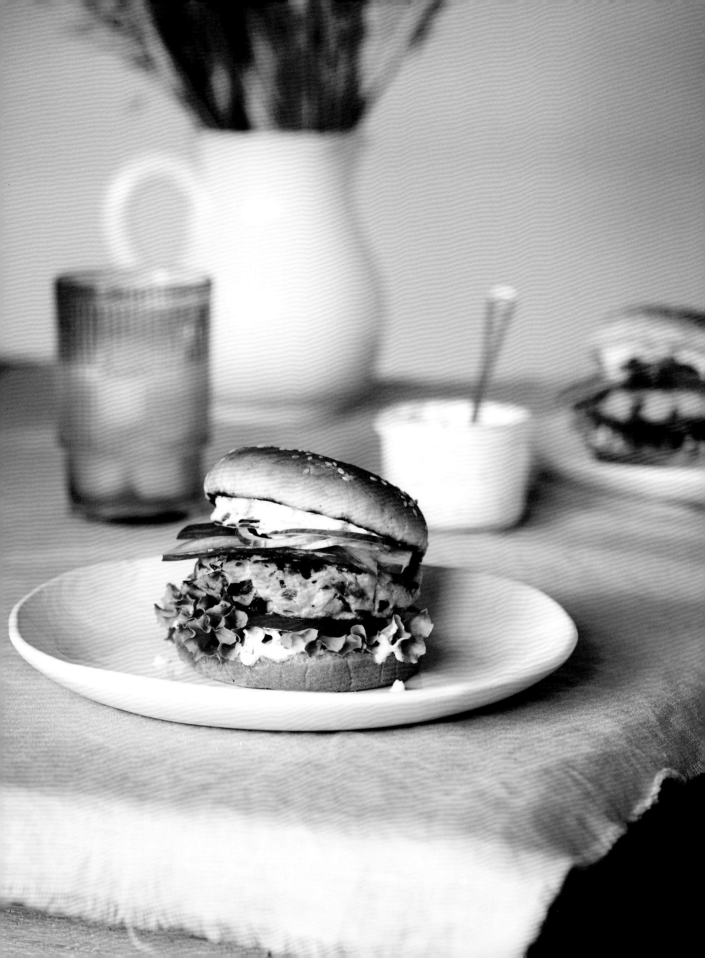

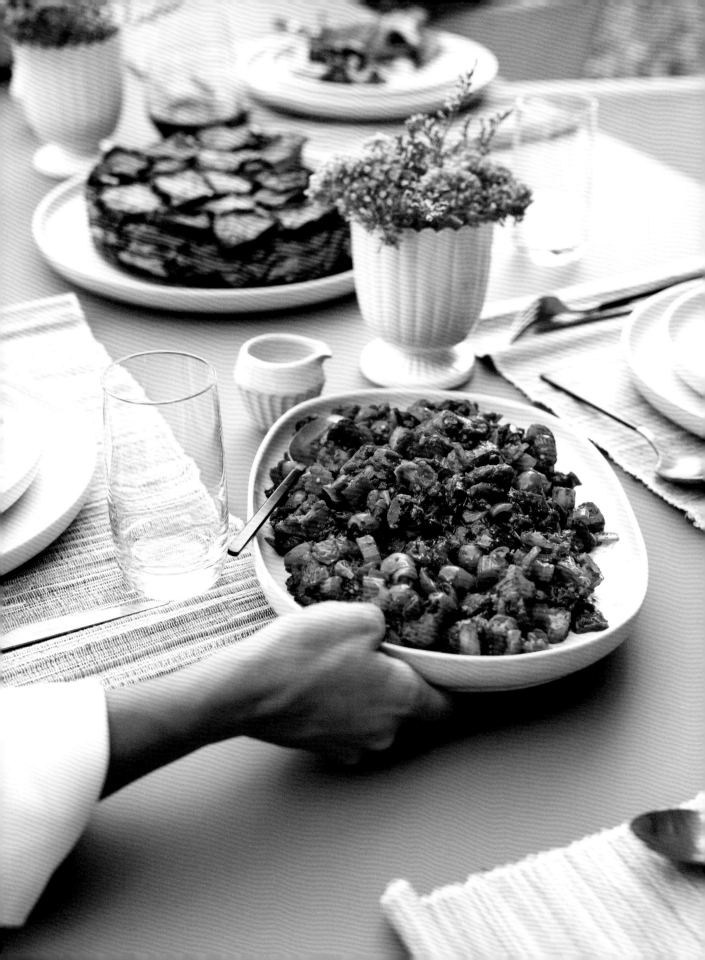

Sunday Gathering

Most of the recipes in this book are great for everyday cooking. But this book would not be faithful to the Mediterranean way without including dishes that require more mindfulness, time, and love, such as those in the following pages, meant to share over leisurely Sunday gatherings that last all afternoon. The menu for such occasions often involves a vegetable-based starter like Caponata (page 210), a pasta dish such as the Eggplant Pasta Bake (page 217), and, sometimes, a braised meat, like the Blade Roast with Parsnips and Shallots (page 220).

Caponata

Vegetarian · Dairy-free · Gluten-free · Nut-free

Caponata is an emblematic Sicilian dish that I grew up eating and that helped cultivate my love of vegetables. It is a sweet and sour cooked salad that celebrates eggplant, onion, and celery, and it can be eaten with absolutely anything: bread, crackers, fish, lamb, on a spoon! Every family has their version. Here is mine, and now yours. MAKES ABOUT 3 CUPS (750 ML)

4 Tbsp (60 mL) olive oil, divided

2 eggplant, cut into 1-inch (2.5 cm) cubes (about 8 cups/2 L)

4 cups (1 L) diced onion

1 Tbsp (15 mL) tomato paste

1 can (14 oz/398 mL) diced tomatoes

2 cups (500 mL) sliced celery (½ inch/1.2 cm thick)

1 cup (250 mL) pitted green olives, halved

3 Tbsp (45 mL) capers

2 Tbsp (30 mL) white wine vinegar

2 Tbsp (30 mL) honey

Salt

1. Heat 2 Tbsp (30 mL) oil in a 12-inch (30 cm) skillet set over medium-high heat. Add the eggplant and cook, stirring frequently, until golden and softened, about 5 minutes. Transfer to a plate.

2. Reduce the heat to medium and add the remaining 2 Tbsp (30 mL) oil. Stir in the onion and tomato paste, then cook for 10 minutes or until the onion is translucent.

3. Return the eggplant to the skillet, and add the tomatoes, celery, olives, capers, vinegar, and honey. Season with salt to taste. Stir and simmer, uncovered, for 15 minutes. The celery should still have bite.

4. Let cool to room temperature before serving. Any leftovers can be stored in an airtight container in the refrigerator for up to 1 week.

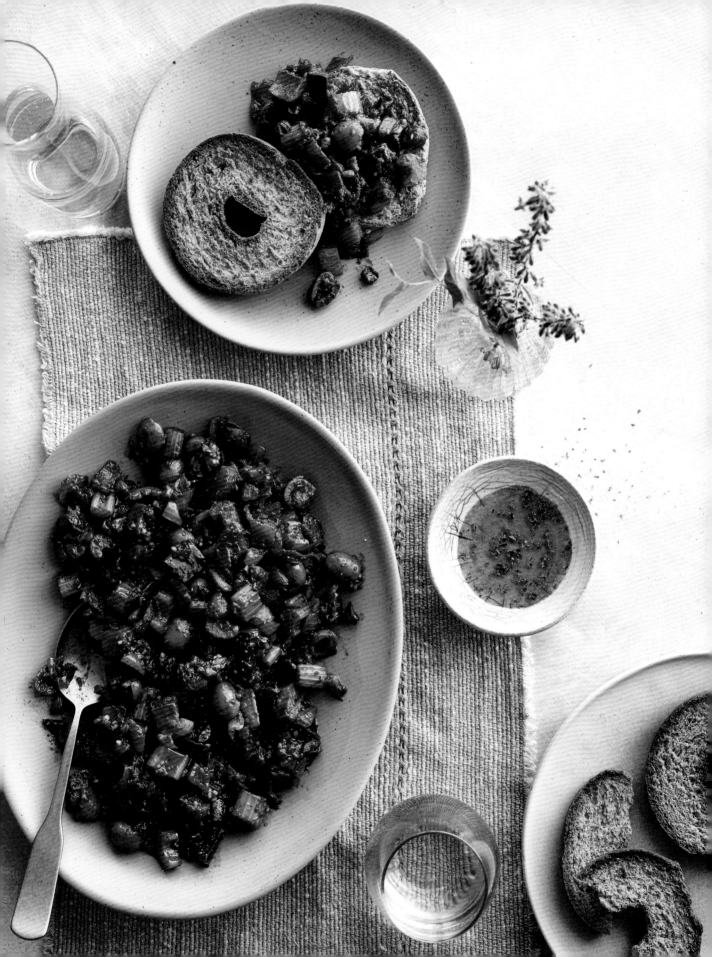

Grilled Octopus with Red Pepper and Caper Relish

Vegetarian · Dairy-free · Gluten-free · Nut-free

Go to any Mediterranean restaurant and you will find a grilled octopus starter on the menu. Here's why I love preparing this dish for guests: it's colorful, elegant, and always popular. The trick to tender grilled octopus is simmering it first, a step I like to do the day before, so that all that's left to do when guests arrive is grill the octopus and top it with the sweet and sour red pepper, caper, and vinegar relish, which can also be made in advance. You will both impress yourself and wow a crowd with this dish. SERVES 6 TO 8

FOR THE OCTOPUS

2 lb (1 kg) octopus legs (thawed if frozen) (see Kitchen Tip)

2 cups (500 mL) dry red wine

1 Tbsp (15 mL) peppercorns

2 bay leaves

Peel of ½ lemon

Salt

Extra virgin olive oil

FOR THE RELISH

1 Tbsp (15 mL) olive oil

1 yellow onion, finely diced

1 red bell pepper, diced

Salt and pepper

2 Tbsp (30 mL) balsamic vinegar

¼ cup (60 mL) chopped fresh flat-leaf parsley

3 Tbsp (45 mL) capers

1. **PREPARE THE OCTOPUS** Place the octopus, wine, peppercorns, bay leaves, and lemon peel in a large pot with enough water to cover the octopus by 2 inches (5 cm). Add a generous pinch of salt. Bring to a boil, then reduce to a gentle simmer. Cook, uncovered, for 1½ hours or until a knife can easily cut into the flesh. Drain and discard the aromatics.

2. Using a knife, slice the octopus into ½-inch (1.2 cm) pieces. Drizzle with olive oil and set aside. (At this point, you can store the cooked octopus in an airtight container in the refrigerator for up to 2 days.)

3. Heat a well-oiled grill pan over high heat. Grill the octopus pieces for 2 to 3 minutes per side, until grill marks appear. Set aside on a plate.

4. **MAKE THE RELISH** Heat the oil in a 10-inch (25 cm) non-stick skillet set over medium heat. Add the onion and bell pepper and cook for 7 minutes or until softened. Add salt and pepper to taste and the vinegar, and allow it to reduce for 1 minute. Transfer the mixture to a small bowl and stir in the parsley and capers. Serve with the octopus. Any leftover octopus can be stored in an air-tight container in the refrigerator for up to 24 hours. Any leftover relish can be stored in an airtight container in the refrigerator for up to 3 days.

KITCHEN TIP: Grilled octopus doesn't have to be reserved for restaurant outings. This dish is proof of that! That said, you can skip the entire first step of this recipe and ask your local fishmonger for pre-cooked octopus legs.

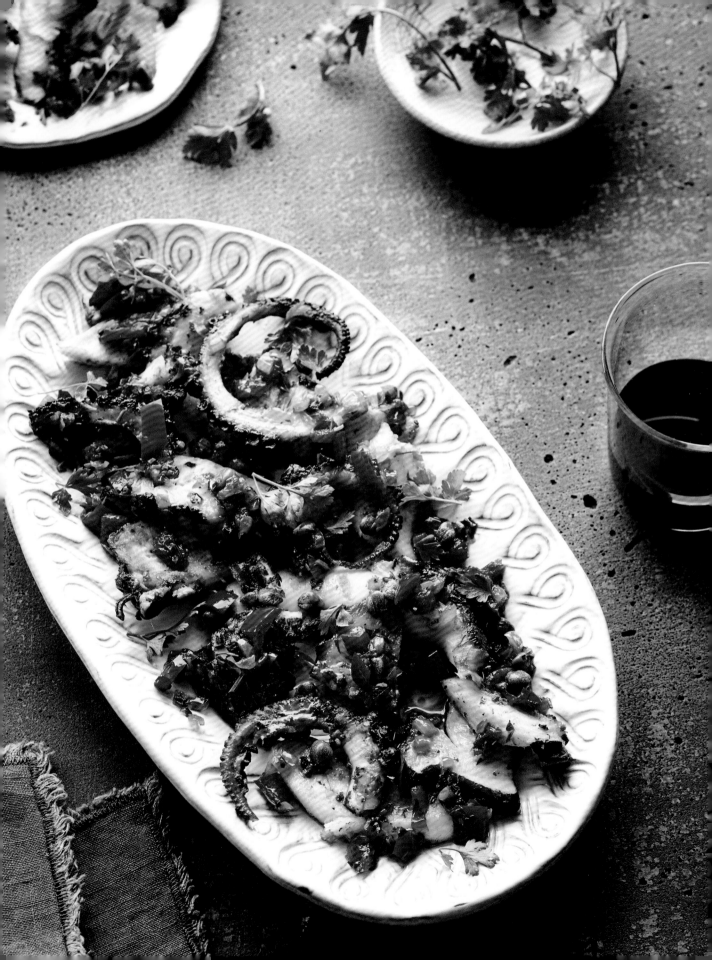

Butternut Squash Lasagna

Vegetarian • Gluten-free • Nut-free

No meal says "family" quite like lasagna. When I was growing up, it was reserved for holidays because of the work involved in making the pasta noodles from scratch. So I was determined to create a vegetable-rich version enjoyed by my entire family, including my son, who has a severe wheat allergy. In this dish, fiber-rich butternut squash is sliced into sheets and layered with a creamy ricotta and spinach filling, then topped with a flavorful tomato sauce. This lasagna is deeply comforting and delicious, and has now earned a spot among the classics in my household. SERVES 6

FOR THE SQUASH NOODLES

2 butternut squash (1 lb/450 g each), peeled

2 Tbsp (30 mL) olive oil

Salt

FOR THE SAUCE

2 Tbsp (30 mL) olive oil

1 yellow onion, finely diced

2 garlic cloves, sliced

1 can (28 oz/796 mL) whole peeled tomatoes

Salt and pepper

½ cup (125 mL) fresh basil

FOR THE LASAGNA

1 cup (250 mL) ricotta

1 cup (250 mL) frozen chopped spinach, thawed and pressed of excess water

¼ cup (60 mL) grated Parmigiano Reggiano

1½ cups (375 mL) grated mozzarella

1. Preheat the oven to 375°F (190°C). Line two baking sheets with parchment paper.

2. **PREPARE THE SQUASH NOODLES** Using a sharp knife, trim the ends of the squash and then cut it in half lengthwise. Remove the seeds using a spoon. Cut the squash in two, where the bulb meets the neck. This will make for easier slicing, as you will have one rectangular piece and one semi-circle.

3. Using a mandoline (set at ⅛ inch/3 mm) or a sharp knife, slice the squash evenly.

4. Place the squash on the prepared baking sheets, brush with the oil, and sprinkle with the salt. Bake for 15 minutes or until tender but still holding their shape. Set aside but keep the oven turned on.

5. **MAKE THE SAUCE** While the squash is baking, heat the oil in a large saucepan set over medium-high heat. Add the onion and cook for 5 minutes or until softened. Add the garlic and cook for 1 minute or until fragrant. Stir in the tomatoes and salt and pepper to taste, then bring to a boil. Reduce to a simmer, cover, and cook for 20 minutes. Add the basil and adjust the seasoning to taste. Let cool.

6. **PREPARE THE LASAGNA** In a bowl, combine the ricotta, spinach, and parmesan.

recipe continues

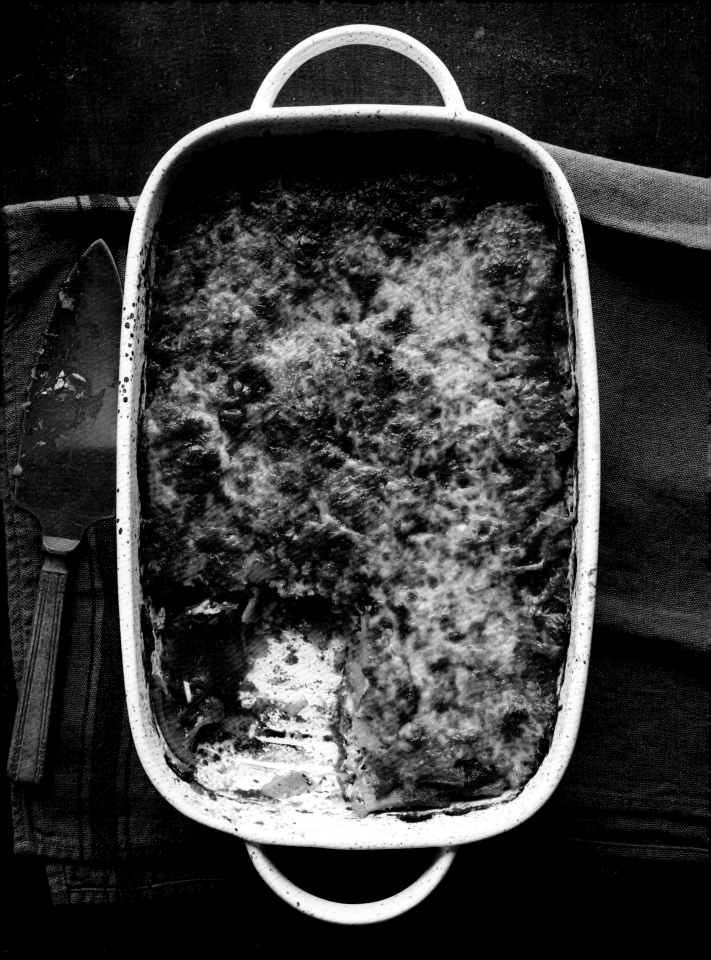

7. Spread a ladle of sauce in the bottom of a 9 × 13-inch (23 × 33 cm) baking dish. Place an even layer of squash, followed by another layer of sauce, then dollop on, here and there, half of the ricotta filling. Repeat with the remaining ingredients, ending with the sauce. Cover the baking dish with aluminum foil and bake for 45 minutes. Remove the aluminum foil, sprinkle with the mozzarella, and return to the oven for 10 minutes or until the cheese is melted. Let rest for 15 minutes before serving. Any leftovers can be stored in an airtight container in the refrigerator for up to 3 days or in the freezer for up to 3 months.

Eggplant Pasta Bake

Vegetarian • Nut-free

I can't help but smile when I think of this dish, as for me it's synonymous with al fresco dining and luncheoning in late summer, when eggplant is at its peak. Eggplant is a quintessential Mediterranean vegetable, and a very good source of dietary fiber and anthocyanins—antioxidant-rich pigments responsible for its deep purple skin. Eggplant pairs wonderfully with tomato, so naturally that combination works well in pasta dishes like this one. This eggplant pasta bake can be entirely prepared in advance, and served hot or warm. SERVES 6

1. Adjust the oven rack to the top position and preheat the oven to broil. Line a baking sheet with parchment paper.

2. Spread the eggplant slices on the prepared baking sheet. Brush both sides with some extra virgin olive oil, and season with salt and pepper. Broil for 10 to 12 minutes, until golden and softened, turning halfway through.

3. Heat the oil in a large saucepan set over medium heat. Add the onion and cook for 5 minutes or until softened. Add the garlic and hot pepper, and cook for 1 minute or until fragrant. Stir in the tomato purée and 1 cup (250 mL) water measured from the empty tomato purée jar, rinsing it of any remaining purée. Add the basil and salt and pepper to taste. Bring to a boil, then reduce to a simmer and cook for 15 to 20 minutes to allow the flavors to meld.

4. Bring a large pot of salted water to a boil and cook the penne according to the package directions. Drain and toss with 2 cups (500 mL) sauce, saving the remainder for serving.

5. Preheat the oven to 350°F (180°C). Grease a 10-inch (25 cm) springform pan with olive oil.

2 large eggplant, sliced into ½-inch-thick (1.2 cm) discs (about 30 total)

Salt and pepper

1 Tbsp (15 mL) extra virgin olive oil

1 onion, diced

2 garlic cloves, sliced

1 red Italian Long Hot pepper, thinly sliced

1 jar (24 oz or 680 mL) tomato purée (passata)

1 cup (250 mL) water

1 cup (250 mL) fresh basil

3 cups (750 mL) penne

½ cup (125 mL) grated Parmigiano Reggiano

1 ball (7 oz/200 g) fresh mozzarella, sliced

recipe continues

6. Place half of the eggplant in a layer in the prepared springform pan, trying to fill any gaps. Top with the pasta, parmesan, and mozzarella, and then with another layer of eggplant. Place the pan on a baking sheet. Bake for 20 to 25 minutes, until the cheese is melted. Let cool for 15 minutes before unmolding.

7. Slice into wedges using a serrated knife. Serve with the remaining sauce, if desired. Any leftovers can be stored in an airtight container in the refrigerator for up to 3 days or in the freezer for up to 3 months.

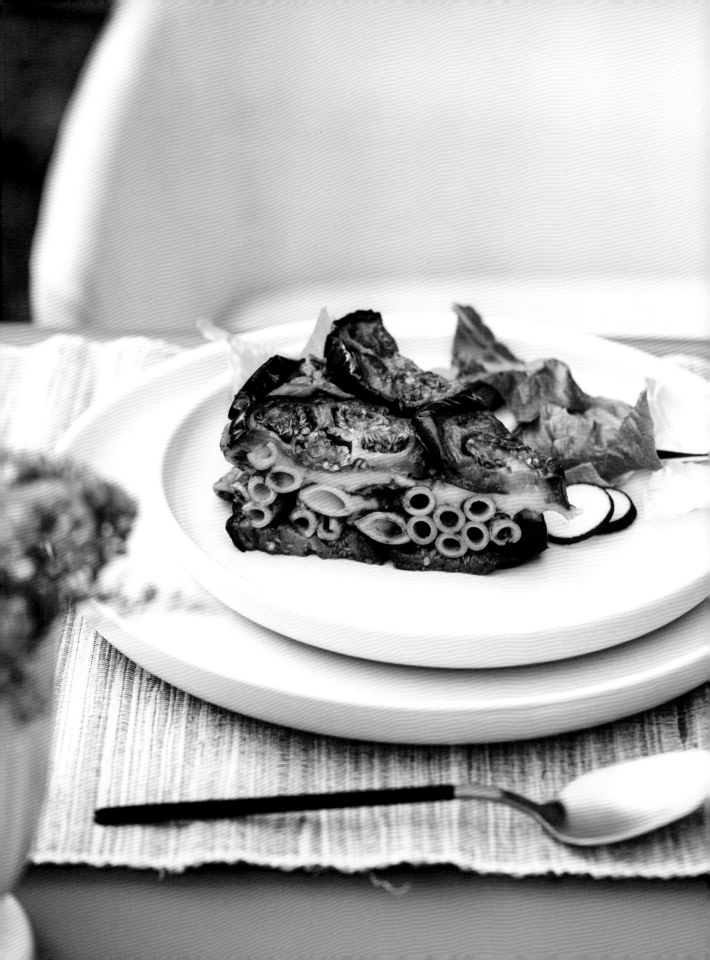

Blade Roast with Parsnips and Shallots

Dairy-free • Gluten-free • Nut-free

This classic set-it-and-forget-it meal is ideal for a Sunday afternoon and makes an impressive main, using simple ingredients. This meaty dish is paired with sweet parsnips and plenty of shallots, a humble vegetable from the allium family (that also includes garlic and onions) that offers up lots of flavor, fiber, and health-protective properties, thanks to its sulfur content. Enjoy this roast with crusty bread, or coarsely shred the meat with a fork and serve with tagliatelle. SERVES 8

1 boneless beef blade roast
    (3 lb/1.5 kg)

Salt and pepper

2 Tbsp (30 mL) olive oil, divided

1 yellow onion, chopped

1 cup (250 mL) dry red wine

½ cup (125 mL) beef broth

½ cup (125 mL) tomato purée
    (passata)

3 Tbsp (45 mL) tomato paste

4 bay leaves

3 sprigs of thyme

10 shallots, halved lengthwise

6 parsnips, peeled and cut into
    2-inch-long (5 cm) pieces

1. Preheat the oven to 325°F (165°C).

2. Season the meat well with salt and pepper on all sides.

3. Heat 1 Tbsp (15 mL) oil in a large Dutch oven set over medium-high heat. Brown the meat on all sides, then transfer to a plate.

4. Reduce the heat to medium and add the remaining 1 Tbsp (15 mL) oil. Add the onion and cook for 3 minutes or until softened. Add the wine, broth, tomato purée, tomato paste, bay leaves, and thyme. Add a good pinch of salt, stir to mix, and then return the meat to the pan. Arrange the shallots and parsnips around the meat.

5. Cover and roast for 3 hours, until the meat easily flakes with a fork. Adjust the seasoning to taste and serve. Any leftovers can be stored in an airtight container in the refrigerator for up to 3 days or in the freezer for up to 3 months.

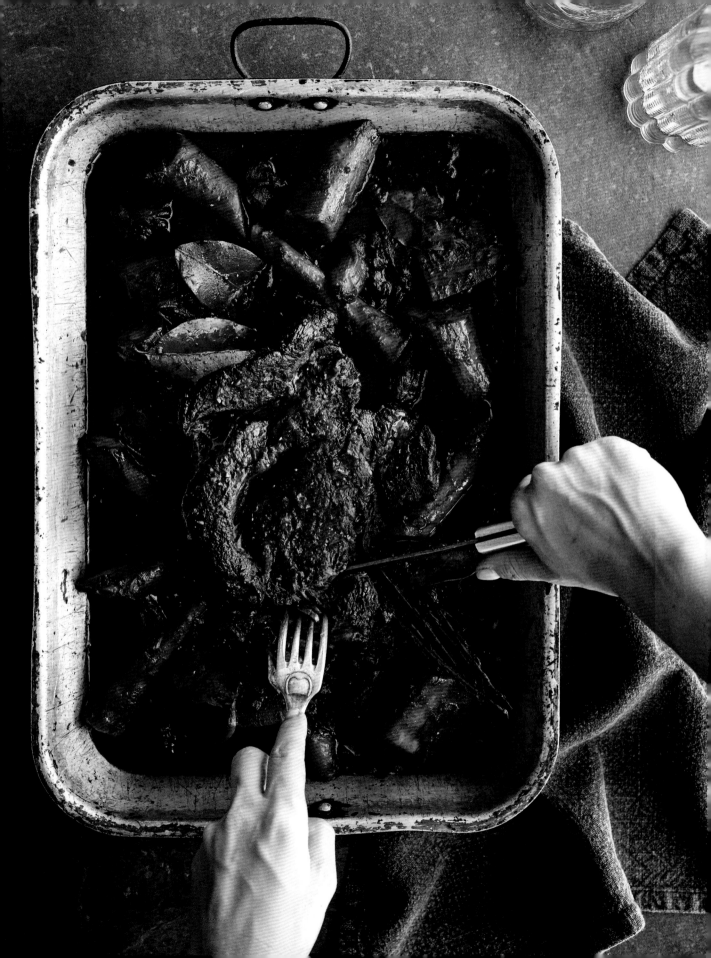

Lamb Stew with Tomatoes, Raisins, and Israeli Couscous

Dairy-free • Nut-free

The Sicilian flavors from the sweet raisins and briny capers pair wonderfully with the lamb in this dish. Keeping with the principles of the Mediterranean diet, this is a dish that would be reserved for special occasions, seeing that meat is the main ingredient. I love that the couscous in this dish cooks directly in the stew, making it a simple one-pot meal—an added bonus for easy entertaining. SERVES 8

2 lb (1 kg) boneless lamb shoulder, cubed

Salt and pepper

2 Tbsp (30 mL) olive oil, divided

2 cups (500 mL) diced onion

4 garlic cloves, minced

2 Tbsp (30 mL) tomato paste

¾ cup (180 mL) dry white wine

4 Roma tomatoes, diced

¼ cup (60 mL) golden raisins

2 Tbsp (30 mL) capers

3 cups (750 mL) low-sodium beef broth

3 sprigs of rosemary

1 cup (250 mL) Israeli couscous

1. Preheat oven to 350°F (180°C).

2. Season the lamb well with salt and pepper.

3. Heat 1 Tbsp (15 mL) oil in a large Dutch oven set over medium-high heat. Brown the lamb on all sides, about 5 minutes. Transfer to a plate.

4. Reduce the heat to medium and add the remaining 1 Tbsp (15 mL) oil. Add the onion and cook for 5 minutes or until softened. Add the garlic and tomato paste, stirring to coat. Deglaze with the wine and reduce, 1 minute. Add the tomatoes, raisins, and capers, followed by the broth and rosemary. Season with salt and pepper, return the lamb to the Dutch oven, stir, and cover.

5. Cook in the preheated oven for 45 minutes or until the meat is fork-tender.

6. Add the couscous to the stew, stir, and return to the oven for 20 minutes or until the couscous is cooked through. Adjust the seasoning to taste and serve. Any leftovers can be stored in an airtight container in the refrigerator for up to 3 days or in the freezer for up to 3 months.

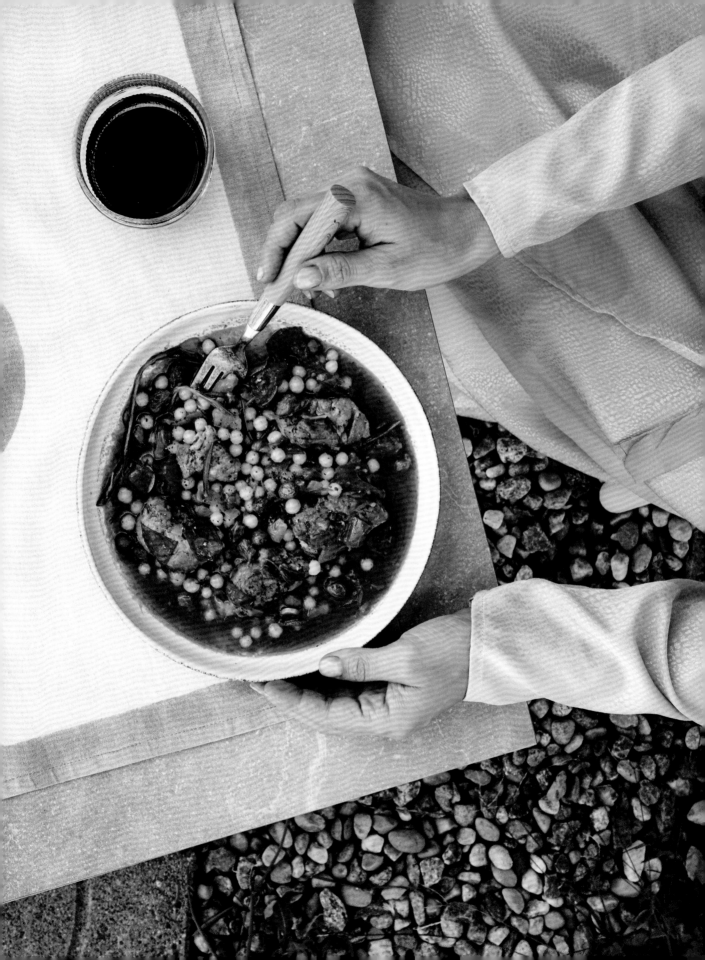

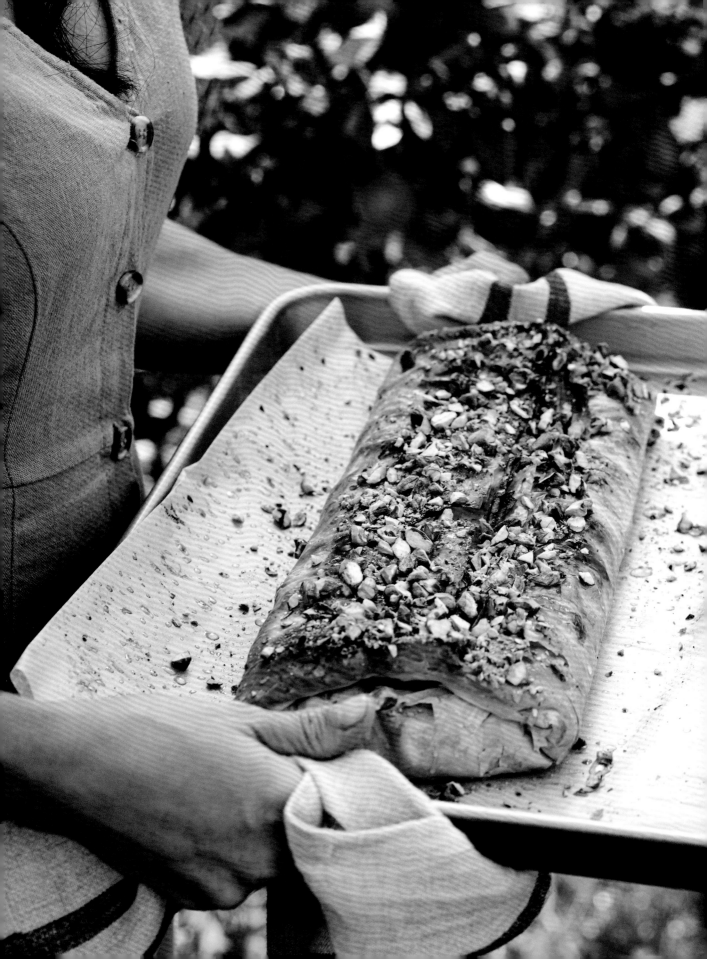

Sweets and Desserts

Mediterranean desserts have a way of being unpretentious, comforting, and delightful all at once. This chapter is filled with inspiration for sweetening your special occasions, whether you wish to end a dinner party with a slice of the Flourless Chocolate, Hazelnut, and Espresso Cake (page 226) or serve Chocolate Chip and Almond Cantuccini (page 228) for an afternoon espresso visit. Some of the recipes in this chapter have been developed to be gluten-free, and when possible, I've included high-fiber alternatives. I hope you explore the delicious options made with nuts, cornmeal, and more!

Flourless Chocolate, Hazelnut, and Espresso Cake

Vegetarian · Gluten-free · Dairy-free

Chocolate lovers rejoice—this one's for you. This flourless cake is inspired by the classic Caprese torte and is made from fiber-rich hazelnuts, pulsed into a flour for an almost brownie-like dessert. I like to add a hint of espresso powder, as it enhances the flavor of this cake beautifully—coffee is an always-welcome pairing with chocolate. SERVES 10 TO 12

1½ cups (375 mL) skinless hazelnuts, plus 2 Tbsp (30 mL) to garnish (optional) (see Kitchen Tip)

1 cup (250 mL) semi-sweet chocolate chips

½ cup (125 mL) extra virgin olive oil

1½ Tbsp (22 mL) espresso powder

4 eggs, separated

¾ cup (180 mL) sugar

¼ tsp (1 mL) salt

2 Tbsp (30 mL) cocoa powder

1. Preheat the oven to 350°F (180°C). Grease a 9-inch (23 cm) springform pan and line the bottom with parchment paper.

2. In a food processor fitted with a steel blade, grind the hazelnuts until they resemble a coarse meal.

3. Melt the chocolate in the microwave, slowly, at 20-second intervals. Once melted, whisk in the oil and espresso powder. Let cool to room temperature.

4. In a large bowl and using an electric mixer, beat the egg yolks with the sugar on high speed for 5 minutes or until pale yellow and airy. Add the chocolate mixture and ground hazelnuts and stir to combine, using a rubber spatula.

5. In a clean bowl and using the (cleaned) electric mixer on high speed, beat the egg whites and salt for 2 minutes or until stiff peaks form. Gently fold the whites into the chocolate mixture by mixing from bottom to top.

6. Pour the batter into the prepared pan and bake for 40 to 45 minutes, until the top is firm to the touch.

7. Let cool completely before unmolding. Using a fine-mesh sieve, dust cocoa powder and sprinkle the remaining 2 Tbsp (30 mL) hazelnuts over the cake. Any leftovers can be covered and stored at room temperature for up to 2 days or in the freezer for up to 2 months.

KITCHEN TIP: Hazelnut skins can be quite bitter. If you can't find skinless hazelnuts, here's how to remove the skins at home. Place the hazelnuts on a baking sheet and bake at 375°F (190°C) for 10 to 15 minutes, or until they've darkened slightly. Transfer the roasted hazelnuts to a clean kitchen towel, fold the cloth over them, and rub vigorously to loosen the skins. Most of the skin should come right off, though a small amount may still be adhering, which is okay. Transfer the clean nuts to a bowl and discard the skins.

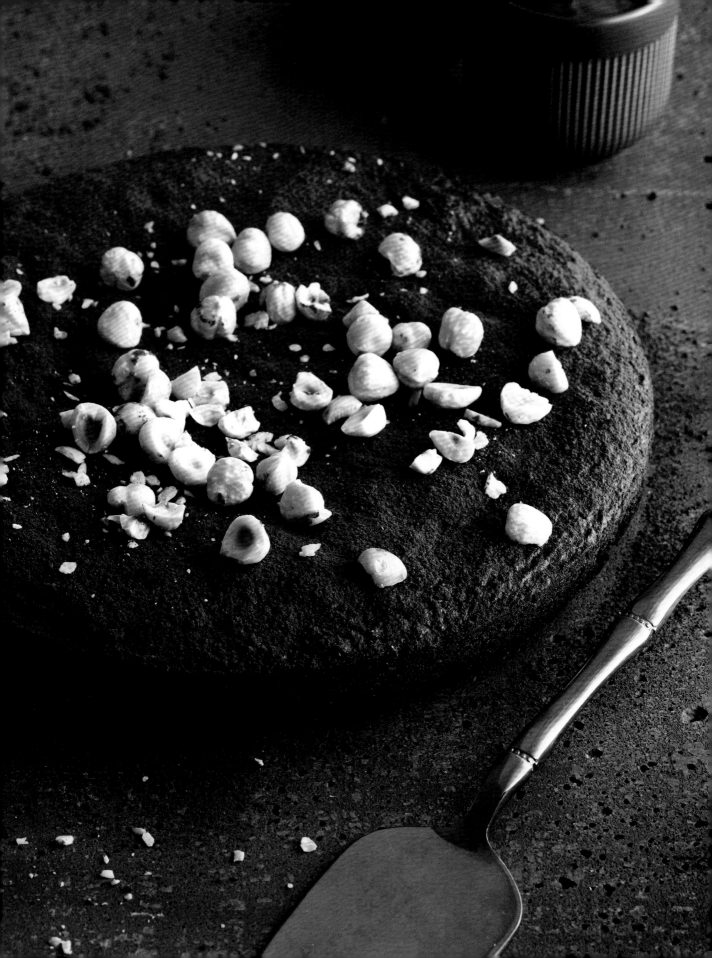

Chocolate Chip and Almond Cantuccini

Vegetarian • Dairy-free

Cantuccini are small cookies typically enjoyed with an espresso or a small glass of Vin Santo. These store beautifully in the freezer and are my go-to sweet for afternoon guests. The spelt flour in this recipe is actually my preference to all-purpose, as it offers a nuttiness to the cookies without tasting "whole wheat-y." MAKES 40 COOKIES

⅔ cup (160 mL) raw whole almonds

2 cups (500 mL) spelt flour

¾ cup (180 mL) sugar

1 tsp (5 mL) baking powder

¼ tsp (1 mL) salt

¼ cup (60 mL) mini semi-sweet chocolate chips

2 eggs

Zest of 1 orange

3 Tbsp (45 mL) olive oil

1 Tbsp (15 mL) honey

1. Preheat the oven to 350°F (180°C). Line a baking sheet with parchment paper.

2. Place the almonds on the prepared baking sheet and toast in the oven for 5 minutes or until fragrant and slightly toasted.

3. In a large bowl, combine the flour, sugar, baking powder, and salt. Add the almonds and chocolate chips, stirring to combine. Reserve the baking sheet. In another large bowl, whisk together the eggs, orange zest, oil, and honey to combine.

4. Using a wooden spoon, add the wet ingredients to the dry ingredients, stirring together until the flour is moistened. Using floured hands, turn the dough onto a floured work surface and knead the dough just until smooth.

5. Divide the dough into two equal portions, form into logs, and place on the baking sheet. Flatten each log so that it is about 1 inch (2.5 cm) wide and ½ inch (1.2 cm) thick.

6. Bake for 20 minutes or until golden. Let cool. Reduce the oven temperature to 325°F (165°C).

7. Gently transfer the logs to a cutting board, reserving the baking sheet. Using a sharp knife, cut into ½-inch-thick (1.2 cm) slices. Lay the cookies flat on the baking sheet.

8. Bake for 12 minutes or until golden brown, turning the cookies halfway through. Let cool. Store in an airtight container at room temperature for up to 1 week or in the freezer for up to 3 months.

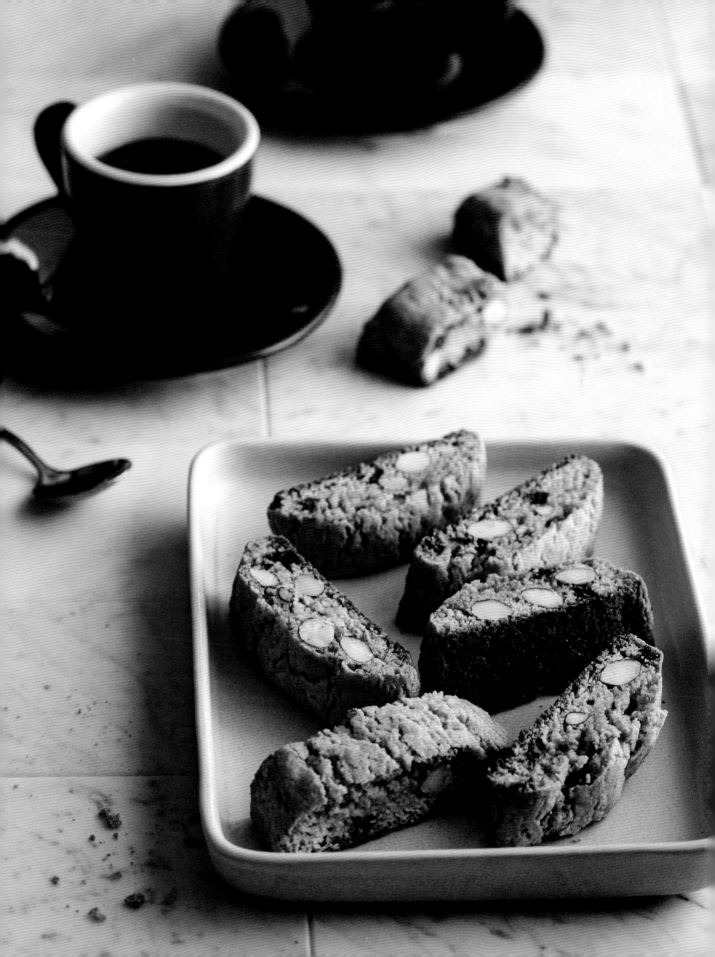

Orange, Polenta, and Olive Oil Cake

Vegetarian • Dairy-free • Gluten-free

This cake is a twist on my family's classic polenta cake. Since I know adding fruit purées to a cake batter can help reduce sugar content without compromising flavor, here I'm taking a cue from the technique used in the Sicilian pan d'arancio and puréeing a whole orange (peel and all) and adding it to the mix. The result is a moist cake with intense orange flavor that gets better with time. SERVES 8

1 seedless orange, such as Cara Cara

1 Tbsp (15 mL) + ⅓ cup (80 mL) olive oil, divided

1½ cups (375 mL) almond flour

1 cup (250 mL) fine cornmeal or polenta

2 tsp (10 mL) baking powder

½ tsp (2.5 mL) salt

⅔ cup (160 mL) sugar

3 eggs

1 tsp (5 mL) pure vanilla extract

¼ cup (60 mL) orange marmalade

3 Tbsp (45 mL) hot water

1. Preheat the oven to 350°F (180°C). Grease a 9-inch (23 cm) springform pan and line the bottom with parchment paper.

2. Wash the orange, cut it into quarters, and place it (still peeled) in a blender or food processor fitted with a steel blade. Add 1 Tbsp (15 mL) oil and purée until smooth, 1 to 2 minutes, scraping down the sides of the blender as needed.

3. In a large bowl, combine the almond flour, cornmeal, baking powder, and salt.

4. In a separate large bowl and using an electric mixer, beat the remaining ⅓ cup (80 mL) oil with the sugar on high speed for 2 minutes or until well combined. Add the eggs, one at a time, beating between each addition. Add the orange purée and vanilla, and mix until combined.

5. Using a spatula, incorporate the dry ingredients into the wet ingredients, stirring to combine.

6. Pour the batter into the prepared pan and bake for 30 minutes or until the center of the top springs back to the touch. Let cool completely before unmolding.

7. In a small bowl, combine the marmalade and water. Prick the top of the cake all over with a toothpick, then pour the marmalade syrup over the cake. Serve. Any leftovers can be covered and stored at room temperature for up to 2 days or in the freezer for up to 2 months.

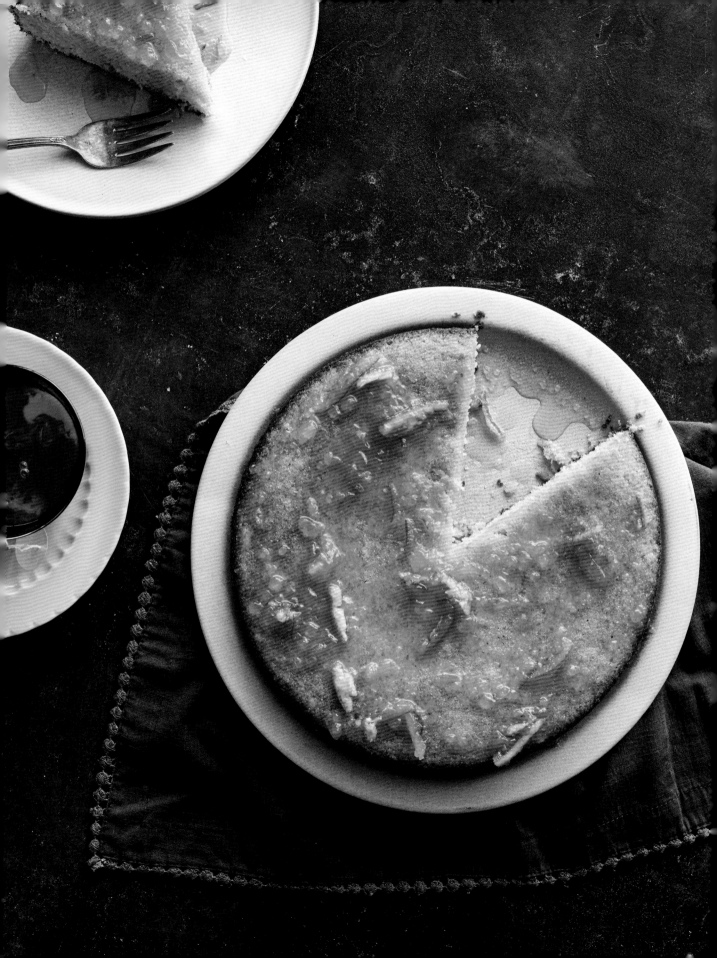

Baklava-Style Apple Strudel

Vegetarian • Dairy-free

Dessert is a wonderful opportunity to celebrate seasonality, a key element of the Mediterranean lifestyle. In Canada, apple season is often synonymous with a trip to the orchard—a fun family tradition resulting in bushels of fruit to take home. This dish is a cross between an apple pie and the classic Mediterranean baklava by using phyllo pastry and combining sweet apples, warming cinnamon, and crunchy nuts. I'm sure this strudel will become your new favorite recipe to welcome the fall. SERVES 8 TO 10

¾ cup (180 mL) raw walnuts

½ cup (125 mL) pistachios

1 tsp (5 mL) ground cinnamon

6 Gala apples, peeled, cored, and diced

2 Tbsp (30 mL) brown sugar

Zest and juice of 1 orange

8 sheets of phyllo dough

¼ cup (60 mL) olive oil

⅓ cup (80 mL) honey, plus more to garnish

1. Preheat the oven to 375°F (190°C).

2. In a food processor fitted with a steel blade, pulse together the walnuts, pistachios, and cinnamon for 15 seconds or until finely chopped. Set aside.

3. In a 12-inch (30 cm) non-stick skillet set over medium heat, sauté the apples, brown sugar, orange zest, and orange juice for 5 minutes, until the apples have tenderized but still have a bite. Pour the cooking juices into a small bowl, and let the apples cool in a separate bowl.

4. Lay the phyllo dough flat on a work surface. Cover with a damp cloth to prevent the sheets from drying.

5. Line a baking sheet with parchment paper. Brush the parchment with a thin layer of oil, then lay the first phyllo sheet on top.

6. Brush the phyllo with about 1 tsp (5 mL) oil, then top with another sheet, pressing firmly with your hands so they stick together. Repeat with the remaining sheets, brushing the last layer with the remaining oil.

7. Reserving 2 Tbsp (30 mL) for garnish, spread the remaining nut mixture onto the phyllo, in an even layer, forming a rectangle in the middle of the phyllo, with a 2-inch (5 cm) border at the bottom and sides and a 3-inch (8 cm) border at the top. Spoon the apple filling over the nuts in an even layer. Pour the honey over the apple filling.

recipe continues

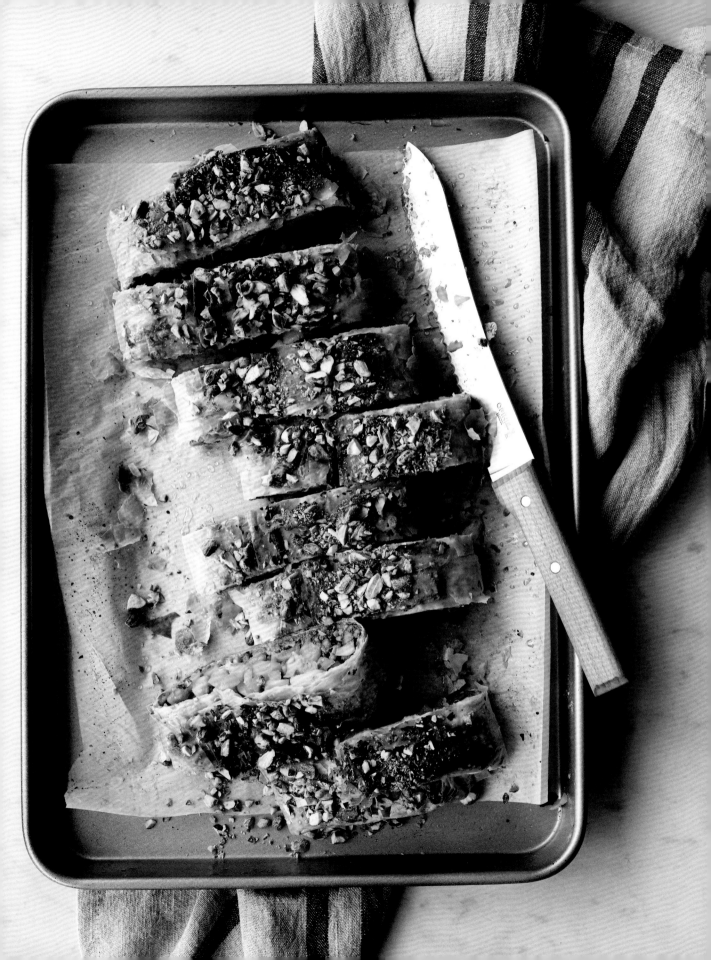

8. Fold the sides of the phyllo rectangle toward the center, covering the mixture, pressing firmly. Brush the folded edges with the reserved apple cooking juices. Fold the bottom of the phyllo rectangle toward the center, covering the mixture, pressing firmly. Brush with the reserved juices. To end, fold the top of the phyllo rectangle toward the center, pressing firmly to seal well. It's important for the seam to be at the top, not underneath the strudel, for even cooking.

9. Brush the top and sides of the strudel with the apple juices and bake for 28 to 30 minutes, or until the top is golden brown.

10. Garnish with a drizzle of honey, and sprinkle with the reserved nut mixture.

11. Carefully transfer to a cutting board using a large spatula. Cut into slices and serve at room temperature (see Kitchen Tip).

KITCHEN TIP: This strudel freezes beautifully. To do this, wrap it tightly in plastic wrap after step 8. Then, when ready to bake, continue with the recipe (step 9). It can be cooked from frozen—simply add an additional 5 minutes to the total cooking time.

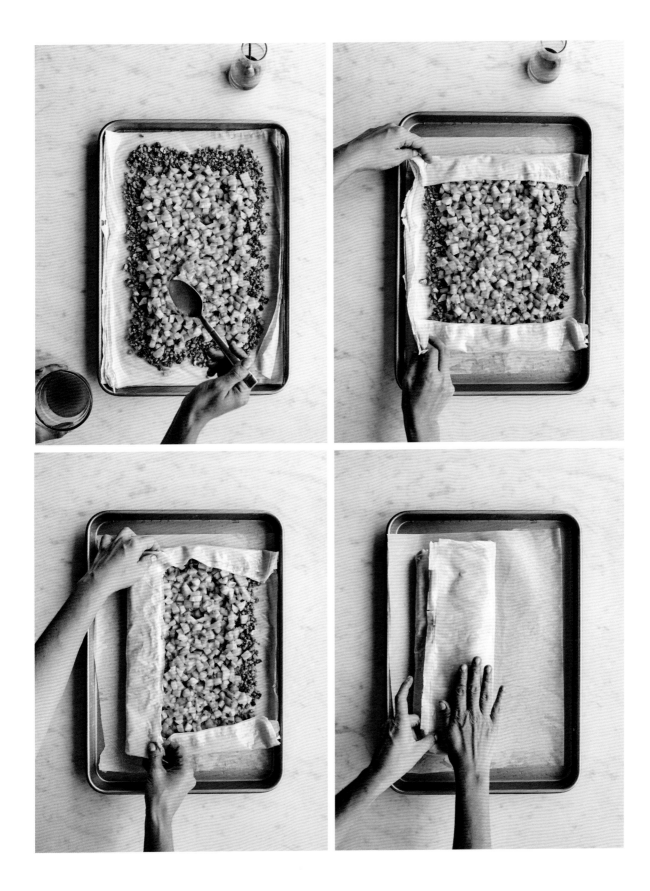

Figgy Walnut Energy Bites

Vegan • Vegetarian • Dairy-free • Gluten-free

When I was younger, my father would prepare fig sandwiches for us after dinner. He would slice dried figs in half and stuff them with so many walnuts you could barely close them shut. Fast-forward to when I met my husband. Turned out that he grew up with the same tradition, except in his version he tucked a small piece of orange peel, which added a lovely citrusy kiss. These energy bites are a quick, satisfying snack inspired by those same flavors. MAKES 10 TO 12 BITES

½ cup (125 mL) whole raw walnuts

¼ cup (60 mL) raw almonds

1 cup (250 mL) dried Kalamata figs, trimmed (see Nutrition Note)

½ tsp (2.5 mL) orange zest

¼ tsp (1 mL) ground cinnamon

2 Tbsp (30 mL) finely chopped raw walnuts

1. In a food processor fitted with a steel blade, pulse the walnuts and almonds until they resemble a coarse meal.

2. Add the figs, orange zest, and cinnamon and process until the mixture pulls away from the sides of the bowl. The dough should stick when pinched between your fingers.

3. Place the chopped walnuts in a small bowl. Using a tablespoon measure, scoop the dough and form into balls, then roll in the chopped walnuts.

4. Store in an airtight container for up to 1 week or in the freezer for up to 3 months.

NUTRITION NOTE: Did you know that dried figs are a high source of calcium? Just eight figs provide over 100 mg of this bone-building nutrient, equivalent to 10% of your daily needs. Eat up!

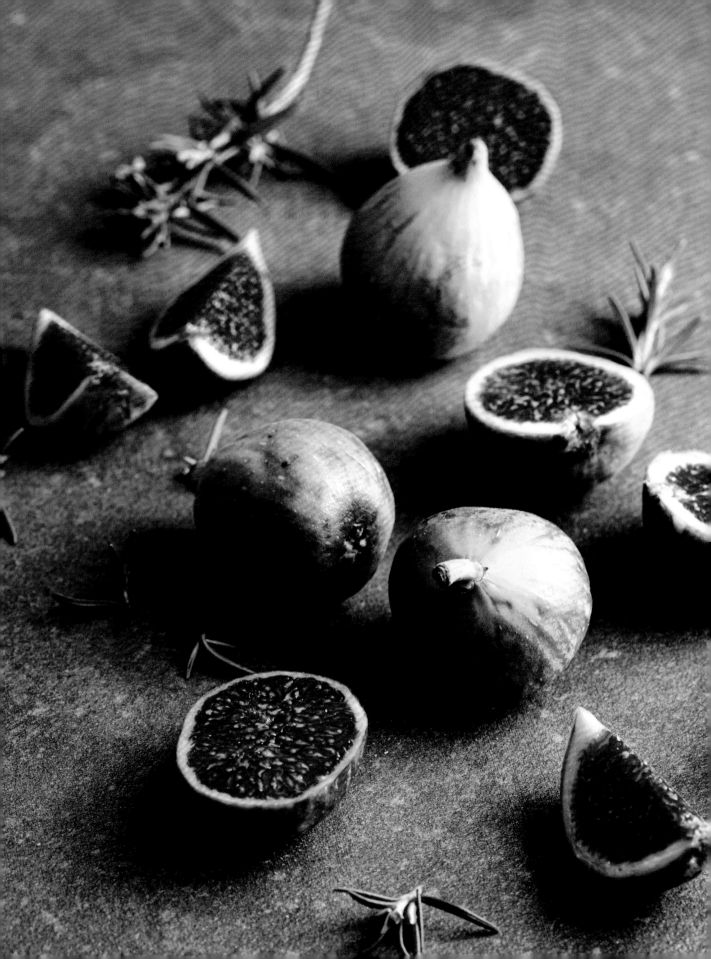

Chewy Hazelnut Bars

Vegetarian • Dairy-free • Gluten-free

These no-bake bars are the ultimate afternoon pick-me-up. The combination of oats, hazelnuts, and hemp seeds provide high-fiber carbohydrates for energy, along with healthy fat and protein to keep energy levels stable in between meals. An added perk is that these bars require no cooking and can be made in advance and stored in the refrigerator or freezer for weekly snacking. MAKES 10 BARS

1 cup (250 mL) certified gluten-free rolled oats

½ cup (125 mL) skinless hazelnuts, chopped

½ cup (125 mL) unsweetened shredded coconut

½ cup (125 mL) dried cherries

¼ cup (60 mL) hemp seeds

2 Tbsp (30 mL) raw cacao powder

Pinch of sea salt

⅓ cup (80 mL) honey

¼ cup (60 mL) hazelnut butter

½ tsp (2.5 mL) pure vanilla extract

1. Line an 8-inch (20 cm) square pan with a long piece of parchment paper, ensuring that the paper is hanging over both sides, to use as a handle.

2. In a large bowl, combine the oats, hazelnuts, coconut, dried cherries, hemp seeds, cacao powder, and salt. Mix to combine.

3. Place the honey, hazelnut butter, and vanilla in a liquid measuring cup and microwave for 30 seconds. Whisk to combine, then pour over the dry ingredients. Stir well to evenly combine.

4. Pour into the prepared pan and press the mixture very firmly into an even layer. Use the excess parchment to press down further. Place in the refrigerator for 4 hours or (preferably) overnight.

5. Use the parchment overhang to remove the slab from the pan. Slice into 10 evenly sized bars. Store in an airtight container in the refrigerator for up to 1 week or in the freezer for up to 2 months.

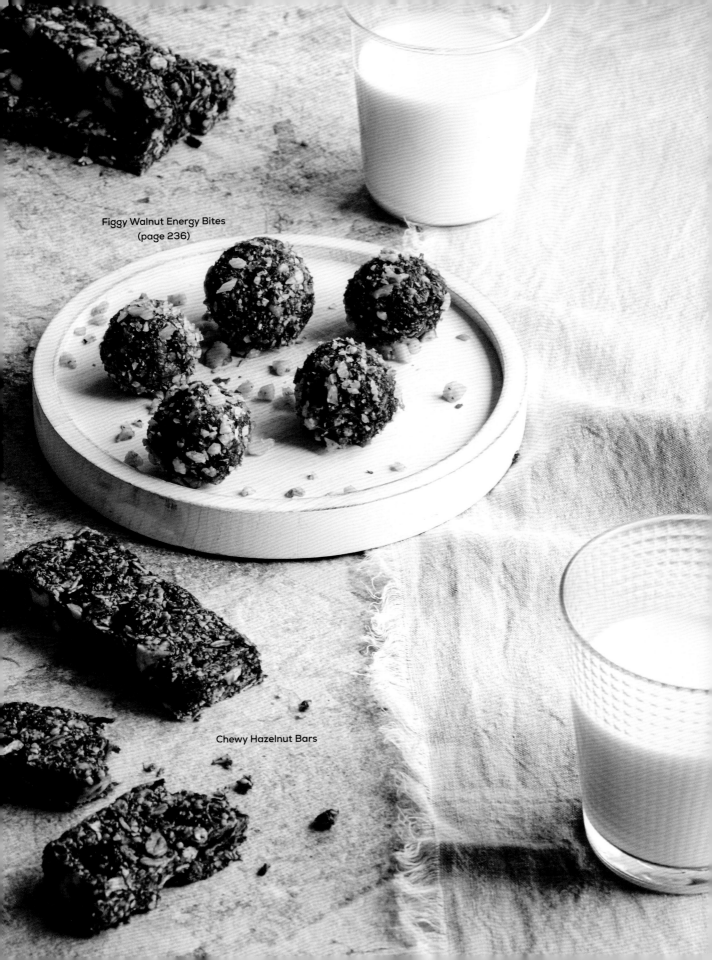

Figgy Walnut Energy Bites
(page 236)

Chewy Hazelnut Bars

No-Bake Honey Yogurt Tart

Gluten-free

This dessert is inspired by one of my favorite Greek treats: yogurt with cherry preserves. Here, I've turned it into a no-fuss gluten-free tart that my little one, who suffers from a severe wheat allergy, can enjoy for dessert. The ingredients are simple and provide a nice blend of fiber, fat, and protein thanks to the combination of fruit, nuts, and Greek yogurt. In fact, it can make for a fun brunch option, as it doesn't read like a traditional dessert. SERVES 6

FOR THE TART

¾ cup (180 mL) certified gluten-free rolled oats

½ cup (125 mL) raw walnuts

1 cup (250 mL) pitted dates

¼ tsp (1 mL) ground cinnamon

1 packet (7 g) gelatin

¼ cup (60 mL) water

¼ cup (60 mL) milk

1¾ cups (430 mL) full-fat Greek yogurt

¼ cup (60 mL) honey

¼ tsp (1 mL) pure vanilla extract

FOR THE COMPOTE

2 cups (500 mL) fresh or frozen cherries, pitted

¼ cup (60 mL) sugar

1 Tbsp (15 mL) water

1 tsp (5 mL) freshly squeezed lemon juice

1. **PREPARE THE TART** In a food processor fitted with a steel blade, grind the oats and walnuts to a coarse meal.

2. Place the dates in a small bowl and cover with hot water. Soak for 5 minutes to tenderize. Drain the dates and add them to the food processor along with the cinnamon. Pulse to obtain a uniform paste that sticks between your fingers.

3. Spread the mixture evenly in a 9-inch (23 cm) springform pan. Use the bottom of a glass to press the crust in firmly.

4. In a small bowl, combine the gelatin and water. Let stand for 5 minutes so that the gelatin can absorb the water. Heat the milk for 30 seconds in the microwave. Add the warm milk to the gelatin mixture, stirring until the gelatin is dissolved.

5. In a large bowl, whisk together the yogurt, honey, and vanilla. Pour in the gelatin mixture, whisking until smooth.

6. Pour the yogurt mixture onto the crust and spread into an even layer. Refrigerate for 8 hours or until the yogurt sets.

7. **PREPARE THE COMPOTE** In a small saucepan set over medium heat, combine the cherries, sugar, water, and lemon juice. Bring to a boil, then reduce to a simmer and cook for 7 to 10 minutes, until the liquid is reduced by one-third. Let the cherries cool to room temperature. Serve with the tart slices. Any leftover compote can be stored in an airtight container in the refrigerator for up to 4 days.

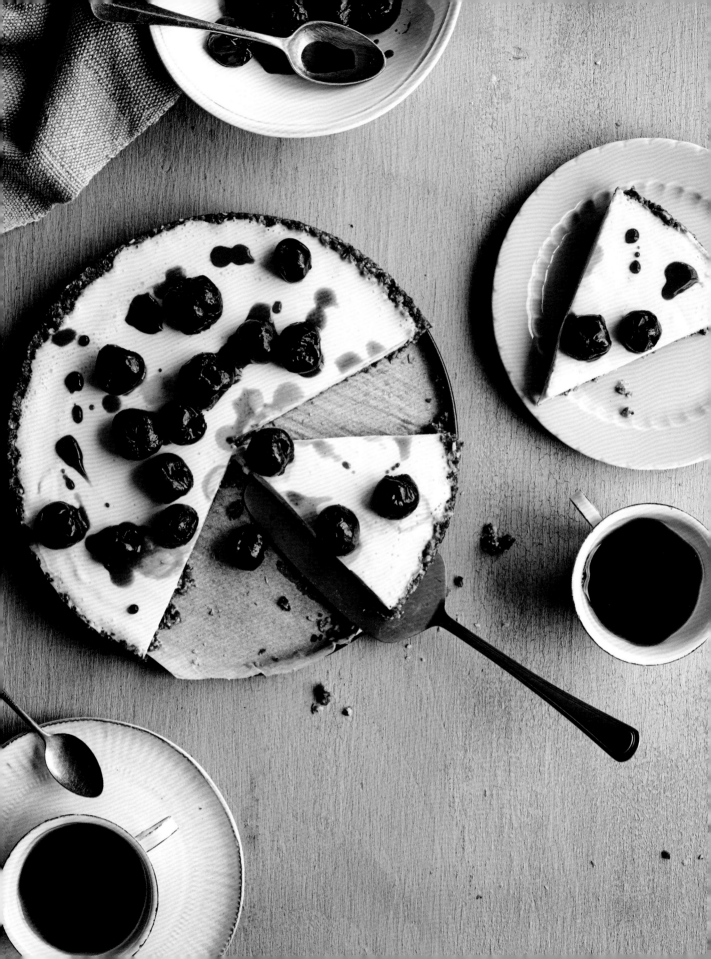

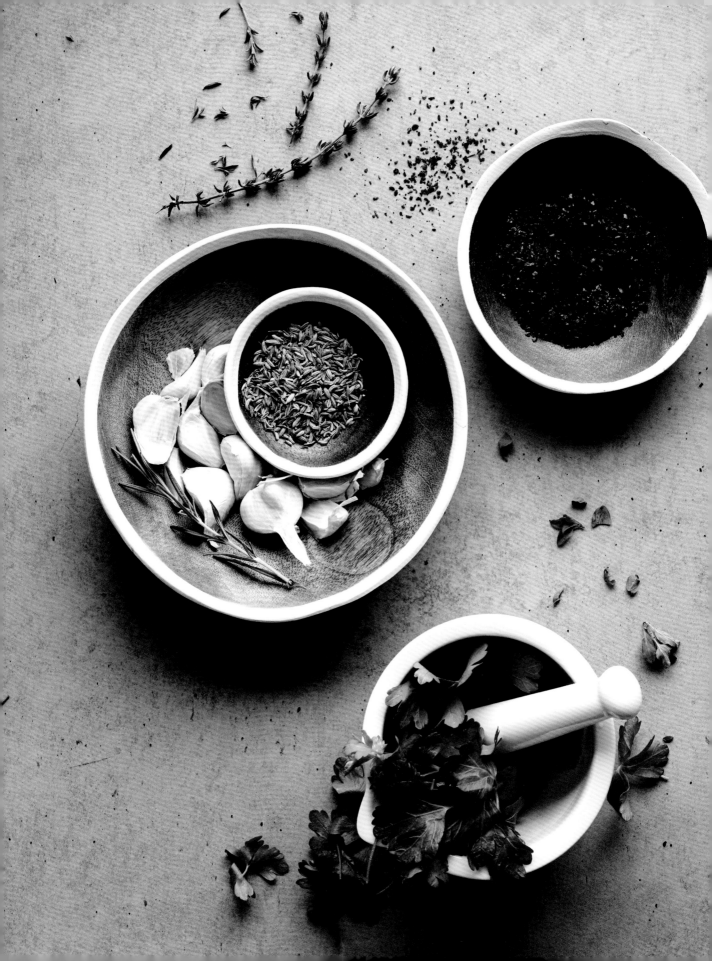

Basics

It's no secret that the way Mediterranean cuisine accomplishes flavorful dishes with simplicity is by seeking out the best ingredients. This often means relying on homemade condiments and pantry staples, like the ones described in this chapter. When making basics like breadcrumbs or pesto at home, you gain control over ingredient quality—and you can taste the difference (plus have the satisfaction of making it from scratch)! That said, store-bought alternatives are also suggested throughout the book; these work well too, especially if you are short on time.

Breadcrumbs

Vegan • Vegetarian • Dairy-free • Nut-free

For such a simple staple, it's surprising that store-bought varieties often have lengthy ingredient lists. Preparing your own breadcrumbs helps keep this staple to one ingredient and is a cost-effective way to use up stale bread. MAKES ABOUT 3 CUPS (750 ML)

1 loaf day-old sourdough bread, crust removed

1. Preheat the oven to 325°F (165°C). Line a baking sheet with parchment paper.

2. Tear the bread into pieces and spread them evenly on the prepared baking sheet.

3. Bake for 25 minutes or until the bread is golden brown and dry. Let cool completely.

4. Transfer to a food processor and pulse into breadcrumbs. Store in an airtight container at room temperature for up to 1 month or in the freezer for up to 3 months. You can use the breadcrumbs directly from the freezer.

SEASONED BREADCRUMBS VARIATION: In a bowl, combine 1 cup (250 mL) plain breadcrumbs (recipe above) with 2 Tbsp (30 mL) finely chopped parsley and 2 Tbsp (30 mL) freshly grated Pecorino Romano. Stir to mix, then store in an airtight container in the freezer for up to 3 months. You can use the breadcrumbs directly from the freezer.

Spice Blends

Spices are liberally used in the Mediterranean diet as flavor enhancers in a variety of dishes. These spice blends are a practical way to jazz up simple meals and last-minute dinners.

Greek Seasoning

Use this spice mix to season chicken, meat, or roast potatoes.

Vegan • Vegetarian • Gluten-free • Dairy-free • Nut-free

2 Tbsp (30 mL) dried oregano

1 Tbsp (15 mL) dried dill

1 Tbsp (15 mL) dried marjoram

1 Tbsp (15 mL) dried thyme

1 tsp (5 mL) granulated garlic

1 tsp (5 mL) granulated onion

1. Place all the ingredients in a bowl and stir to combine. Store in an airtight container in a cool, dry place for up to 6 months.

Makes about ⅓ cup (80 mL)

Herb-Flavored Salt

Use this spice mix to season fish, seafood, or roasted winter squash.

Vegan • Vegetarian • Gluten-free • Dairy-free • Nut-free

1 cup (250 mL) sea salt

1 Tbsp (15 mL) dried parsley

1 Tbsp (15 mL) dried rosemary

1 Tbsp (15 mL) granulated garlic

1 Tbsp (15 mL) freshly cracked pepper

1 tsp (5 mL) dried sage

1. Place all the ingredients in a bowl and stir to combine. Store in an airtight container in a cool, dry place for up to 6 months.

Makes about 1¼ cups (310 mL)

Za'atar

Use this spice mix as a garnish on hummus, yogurt, mixed with extra virgin olive oil for dipping bread, or to season roasted vegetables, salad, meat . . . you name it!

Vegan • Vegetarian • Gluten-free • Dairy-free • Nut-free

2 Tbsp (30 mL) sesame seeds

¼ cup (60 mL) dried oregano

2 Tbsp (30 mL) dried thyme

2 Tbsp (30 mL) sumac

½ tsp (2.5 mL) kosher salt

1. In a small, dry skillet, toast the sesame seeds until fragrant, 3 to 4 minutes. Transfer to a bowl.

2. In a spice grinder, pulse the oregano and thyme. Add to the bowl with the sesame, along with the sumac and salt, and stir to combine. Store in an airtight jar in a cool, dry place for up to 3 months.

Makes about ⅔ cup (160 mL)

Dressings and Marinades

One of the cornerstone ingredients of the Mediterranean diet is quality extra virgin olive oil, known for its unique flavor and healthy fat profile. Making your own dressings and marinades helps you regularly incorporate this beneficial oil into your diet.

Balsamic Vinaigrette

Serve as a salad dressing with bitter greens like radicchio, with the Grilled Vegetables (page 131), or with the Mediterranean Farro and Chickpea Bowl (page 148).

Vegan • Vegetarian • Gluten-free • Dairy-free • Nut-free

¾ cup (180 mL) extra virgin olive oil

¼ cup (60 mL) quality aged balsamic vinegar

½ tsp (2.5 mL) dried oregano

1 garlic clove, halved

Salt and pepper

1. Put the oil, vinegar, oregano, and garlic in a jar, put the lid on tightly, and shake until the dressing is emulsified. Season with salt and pepper and shake again. Remove the garlic before serving. Store in the refrigerator for up to 3 days.

Makes 1 cup (250 mL)

Everyday Dressing

This is my go-to salad dressing. It's the one I prepare when I have a hankering for a big salad, or to drizzle over simple mixed greens, like my Everyday Green Salad (page 136). The flavor is bright and fresh with the vinegar, lemon juice, and mint.

Vegetarian • Gluten-free • Dairy-free • Nut-free

⅔ cup (160 mL) extra virgin olive oil

¼ cup (60 mL) good white wine vinegar (I like Forvm brand)

2 Tbsp (30 mL) freshly squeezed lemon juice

1 Tbsp (15 mL) honey

1 Tbsp (15 mL) Dijon mustard

½ tsp (2.5 mL) dried oregano

½ tsp (2.5 mL) dried mint

1 garlic clove, crushed

Salt and pepper

1. Put the oil, vinegar, lemon juice, honey, mustard, oregano, mint, and garlic in a jar, put the lid on tightly, and shake until the dressing is emulsified. Add salt and pepper to taste and shake again. Remove the garlic clove before serving. Store in the refrigerator for up to 4 days. Remove from the refrigerator 15 minutes before using.

Makes 1 cup (250 mL)

Lemon and Herb Marinade

This marinade pairs well with tofu, shrimp, or chicken.

Vegan • Vegetarian • Gluten-free • Dairy-free • Nut-free

¼ cup (60 mL) olive oil

3 Tbsp (45 mL) lemon juice (about 1 lemon)

1 Tbsp (15 mL) lemon zest (1 lemon)

2 tsp (10 mL) fresh oregano (or ½ tsp/2.5 mL dried)

2 tsp (10 mL) fresh thyme (or ½ tsp/2.5 mL dried)

4 garlic cloves, smashed

Freshly ground black pepper

1. Place all the ingredients in a bowl and mix to combine. Store in an airtight jar in the refrigerator for up to 4 days or in a freezer-safe resealable bag in the freezer for up to 3 months.

Makes about ½ cup (125 mL)

KITCHEN TIP: This recipe makes enough marinade for 1 lb (450 g) protein. Feel free to double this recipe and freeze the other half to use another time.

Smoky Yogurt Marinade

This marinade works well for lamb chops or chicken thighs.

Vegetarian • Gluten-free • Nut-free

½ cup (125 mL) plain yogurt

2 Tbsp (30 mL) olive oil

2 Tbsp (30 mL) red wine vinegar

2 Tbsp (30 mL) fresh thyme

1 Tbsp (15 mL) smoked paprika

1 Tbsp (15 mL) tomato paste

6 garlic cloves, smashed

1. Place all the ingredients in a bowl and mix to combine. Store in an airtight jar in the refrigerator for up to 4 days or in a freezer-safe resealable bag in the freezer for up to 3 months.

Makes about ½ cup (125 mL)

KITCHEN TIP: This recipe makes enough marinade for 1 lb (450 g) protein. Feel free to double this recipe and freeze the other half to use another time.

Garlic and Rosemary Marinade

This is a wonderful marinade for pork or beef, or for massaging into a whole chicken before roasting.

Vegan • Vegetarian • Gluten-free • Dairy-free • Nut-free

¼ cup (60 mL) olive oil

2 Tbsp (30 mL) freshly squeezed lemon juice

2 Tbsp (30 mL) minced fresh rosemary

1 Tbsp (15 mL) Dijon mustard

4 garlic cloves, minced

1. Place all the ingredients in a bowl and mix to combine. Store in an airtight jar in the refrigerator for up to 4 days or in a freezer-safe resealable bag in the freezer for up to 3 months.

Makes about ½ cup (125 mL)

KITCHEN TIP: This recipe makes enough marinade for 1 lb (450 g) protein. Feel free to double this recipe and freeze the other half to use another time.

Marinara Sauce

Vegan • Vegetarian • Gluten-free • Dairy-free • Nut-free

This quick recipe is your go-to when you're in need of a simple and flavorful sauce. Use on pizza, as a dipping sauce, or as a base for other sauces. MAKES ABOUT 3½ CUPS (875 ML)

3 Tbsp (45 mL) olive oil

½ onion, finely diced

3 garlic cloves, halved

Pinch of crushed chili flakes

1 can (28 oz/796 mL) diced tomatoes

8 basil leaves, torn

Salt and pepper

1. Heat the oil in a saucepan set over medium-low heat. Add the onion and cook for 5 minutes or until softened.

2. Add the garlic and chili flakes and stir until fragrant, 1 minute. Stir in the tomatoes, basil, and salt and pepper to taste. Bring to a simmer and cook for 20 minutes to allow the flavors to meld. Adjust the seasoning to taste and serve. Store in an airtight container in the refrigerator for up to 5 days or in the freezer for up to 3 months.

Classic Pesto

Vegetarian • Gluten-free

Of all the condiments, pesto is the one I couldn't live without. I use it as a topping on fish for a quick dinner, as a marinade for shrimp, as a sauce for pasta, or to add flavor to roasted potatoes. MAKES ABOUT 1 CUP (250 ML)

2 garlic cloves, peeled

¼ cup (60 mL) pine nuts

Pinch of salt

¼ cup (60 mL) freshly grated Parmigiano Reggiano

4 cups (1 L) fresh Genovese basil

½ cup (125 mL) extra virgin olive oil

1. In a food processor fitted with a steel blade, pulse the garlic, pine nuts, salt, and parmesan to combine. Add the basil and process until smooth.

2. With the motor running at low speed, drizzle in the oil to obtain a creamy consistency. Adjust the seasoning to taste. Store in an airtight container in the refrigerator for up to 4 days or in the freezer for up to 4 months.

KITCHEN TIP: If serving this pesto with pasta, reserve some of the starchy salted pasta water, then add it, 1 Tbsp (15 mL) at a time, to thin the pesto sauce to your desired consistency.

Tzatziki

Vegetarian · Gluten-free · Nut-free

This sharp and refreshing sauce is ideal for the Pork Souvlaki Pitas (page 192) or as a simple dip for crudité to enjoy any day of the week. MAKES ABOUT 1½ CUPS (375 ML)

1 medium cucumber, grated (skin on)

1½ cups (375 mL) full-fat, plain Greek yogurt

2 garlic cloves, finely minced

2 Tbsp (30 mL) extra virgin olive oil

1½ Tbsp (22 mL) quality white wine vinegar (I like Forvm brand)

Salt and pepper

1. Place the grated cucumber in a clean kitchen towel and wring it well. Place the cucumber in a bowl.

2. Add the yogurt, garlic, oil, vinegar, and salt and pepper to taste. Stir together and serve. Store in an airtight container in the refrigerator for up to 3 days, or in the freezer, in an ice cube tray for single servings, for up to 3 months.

Tahini Sauce

Vegan · Vegetarian · Gluten-free · Dairy-free · Nut-free

Nutty sesame flavor is rounded out with lemon in this creamy sauce, perfect for dressing hearty salads or oven-roasted root vegetables, or drizzled over Oven-Baked Spinach Falafel (page 158). MAKES ABOUT ¾ CUP (180 ML)

⅓ cup (80 mL) tahini

⅓ cup (80 mL) water

Juice of 1 lemon

1 garlic clove

Salt and pepper

1. Process the tahini, water, lemon juice, garlic, and salt and pepper to taste in a blender until completely smooth. Store in an airtight container in the refrigerator for up to 3 days.

Salsa Verde

Vegetarian • Gluten-free • Dairy-free • Nut-free

Fresh herbs, zippy lemon, and briny capers create the perfect sauce to brighten up meat dishes or heavier fish, all while adding a welcome dash of green. Serve with Porchetta-Style Tenderloin with Rapini (page 200) or Flank Steak Salad with Crispy White Beans (page 204). MAKES ABOUT ¾ CUP (180 ML)

2 anchovy filets

1 Tbsp (15 mL) capers

2 garlic cloves

1 cup (250 mL) fresh flat-leaf parsley

¼ cup (60 mL) fresh basil

¼ cup (60 mL) fresh mint

Juice of 1 lemon

½ cup (125 mL) extra virgin olive oil, divided

Salt and pepper

1. In a blender, pulse the anchovies, capers, garlic, parsley, basil, mint, lemon juice, and ¼ cup (60 mL) oil until the herbs are finely chopped.

2. Transfer to a bowl, pour in the remaining ¼ cup (60 mL) oil, season with salt and pepper, stir, and serve. Store in an airtight container in the refrigerator for up to 4 days, or in the freezer, in an ice cube tray for single servings, for up to 3 months.

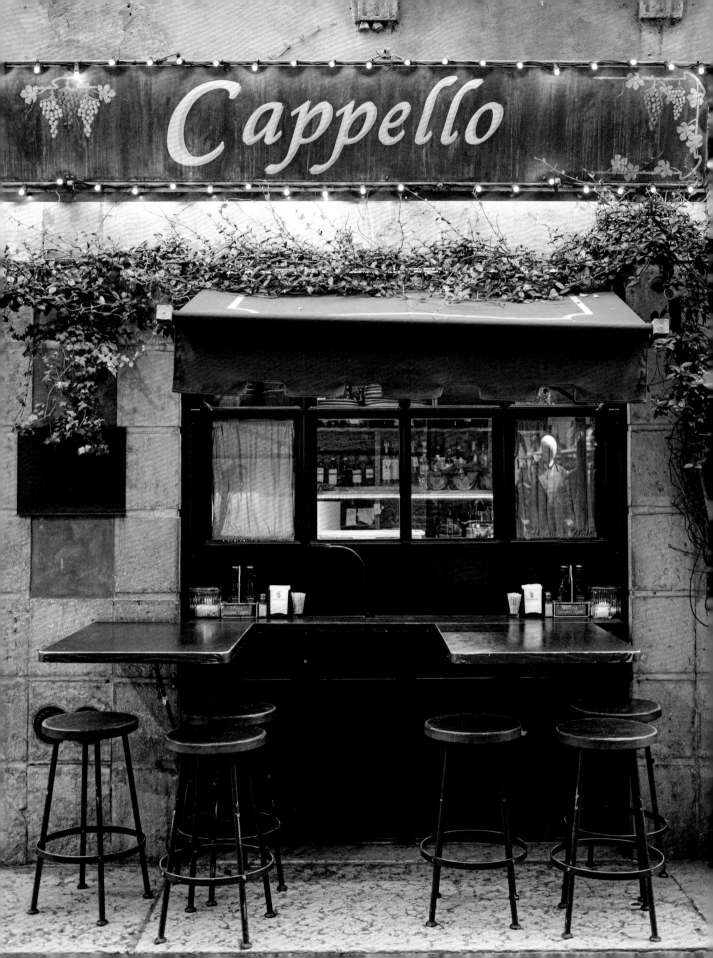

References

Aiello, A., Accardi, G., Caruso, C., Candore, G. 2020. "Effects of Nutraceuticals of Mediterranean Diet on Aging and Longevity." In Preedy, V.R., Watson, R.R., eds., *The Mediterranean Diet*, 2nd ed. Academic Press, 547–53.

Alì, Sawan, et al. 2021. "Healthy Aging and Mediterranean Diet: A Focus on Hormetic Phytochemicals." *Mechanisms of Aging and Development* 200: 111592.

Altomare, Roberta, et al. 2013. "The Mediterranean Diet: A History of Health." *Iranian Journal of Public Health* 42, 5: 449–57.

Bach-Faig, Anna, et al. 2011. "Mediterranean Diet Pyramid Today: Science and Cultural Updates." *Public Health Nutrition* 14, 12A: 2274–84.

Barrea, Luigi, et al. 2019. "Adherence to the Mediterranean Diet, Dietary Patterns and Body Composition in Women with Polycystic Ovary Syndrome (PCOS)." *Nutrients* 11, 10: 2278.

Bonaccio, Marialaura, et al. 2017. "High Adherence to the Mediterranean Diet Is Associated with Cardiovascular Protection in Higher but Not in Lower Socioeconomic Groups: Prospective Findings from the Moli-Sani Study." *International Journal of Epidemiology* 46, 5: 1478–87.

Canudas, Silvia, et al. 2020. "Mediterranean Diet and Telomere Length: A Systematic Review and Meta-Analysis." *Advances in Nutrition* 11, 6: 1544–54.

Cicerale, Sara, et al. 2010. "Biological Activities of Phenolic Compounds Present in Virgin Olive Oil." *International Journal of Molecular Sciences* 11, 2: 458–79.

Davis, Courtney, et al. 2015. "Definition of the Mediterranean Diet: A Literature Review." *Nutrients* 7, 11: 9139–53.

De Alzaa, F., Guillaume, C., and Ravetti, L. 2018. "Evaluation of Chemical and Physical Changes in Different Commercial Oils during Heating." *Acta Scientific* 2, 6: 2–11.

De Lorgeril, M., et al. 1999. "Mediterranean Diet, Traditional Risk Factors, and the Rate of Cardiovascular Complications after Myocardial Infarction: Final Report of the Lyon Diet Heart Study." *Circulation* 99, 6: 779–85.

Dinu, M., et al. 2018. "Mediterranean Diet and Multiple Health Outcomes: An Umbrella Review of Meta-Analyses of Observational Studies and Randomised Trials." *European Journal of Clinical Nutrition* 72, 1: 30–43.

Esposito, Katherine, et al. 2010. "Prevention and Control of Type 2 Diabetes by Mediterranean Diet: A Systematic Review." *Diabetes Research and Clinical Practice* 89, 2: 97–102.

Estruch, Ramón, et al. 2018. "Primary Prevention of Cardiovascular Disease with a Mediterranean Diet Supplemented with Extra-Virgin Olive Oil or Nuts." *New England Journal of Medicine* 378, 25: e34.

Karamanos, B., et al. 2002. "Nutritional Habits in the Mediterranean Basin: The Macronutrient Composition of Diet and Its Relation with the Traditional Mediterranean Diet; Multi-Centre Study of the Mediterranean Group for the Study of Diabetes (MGSD)." *European Journal of Clinical Nutrition* 56, 10: 983–91.

Karayiannis, Dimitrios, et al. 2018. "Adherence to the Mediterranean Diet and IVF Success Rate among Non-obese Women Attempting Fertility." *Human Reproduction* 33, 3: 494–502.

Karayiannis, Dimitrios, et al. 2017. "Association between Adherence to the Mediterranean Diet and Semen Quality Parameters in Male Partners of Couples Attempting Fertility." *Human Reproduction* 32, 1: 215–22.

Keys, A., et al. 1986. "The Diet and 15-Year Death Rate in the Seven Countries Study." *American Journal of Epidemiology* 124, 6: 903–15.

Knoops, Kim T.B., et al. 2004. "Mediterranean Diet, Lifestyle Factors, and 10-Year Mortality in Elderly European Men and Women: The HALE Project." *JAMA* 292, 12: 1433–39.

Lassale, Camille, et al. 2019. "Healthy Dietary Indices and Risk of Depressive Outcomes: A Systematic Review and Meta-Analysis of Observational Studies." *Molecular Psychiatry* 24, 7: 965–86.

Lim, Stephen S., et al. 2012. "A Comparative Risk Assessment of Burden of Disease and Injury Attributable to 67 Risk Factors and Risk Factor Clusters in 21 Regions, 1990-2010: A Systematic Analysis for the Global Burden of Disease Study 2010." *Lancet* 380, 9859: 2224–60.

Linus Pauling Institute. "Phytochemicals." 2022, https://lpi.oregonstate.edu/mic /dietary-factors/phytochemicals

Martínez-González, M.A., et al. 2008. "Adherence to Mediterranean Diet and Risk of Developing Diabetes: Prospective Cohort Study." *BMJ* (Clinical Research ed.) 336, 7657: 1348–51.

Mendonça, Nuno, et al. 2022. "Low Adherence to the Mediterranean Diet Is Associated with Poor Socioeconomic Status and Younger Age: A Cross-Sectional Analysis of the EpiDoC Cohort." *Nutrients* vol. 14, 6: 1239.

Morze, Jakub, et al. 2021. "An Updated Systematic Review and Meta-Analysis on Adherence to Mediterranean Diet and Risk of Cancer." *European Journal of Nutrition* 60, 3: 1561–86.

Nestle, M. 1995. "Mediterranean Diets: Historical and Research Overview." *American Journal of Clinical Nutrition* 61, 6 Suppl: S1313–20.

Papadaki, Angeliki, et al. 2020. "The Effect of the Mediterranean Diet on Metabolic Health: A Systematic Review and Meta-Analysis of Controlled Trials in Adults." *Nutrients* 12, 11: 3342.

Ramseyer Winter, Virginia, et al. 2019. "Eating Breakfast and Family Meals in Adolescence: The Role of Body Image." *Social Work in Public Health* 34, 3: 230–38.

Samieri, Cécilia, et al. 2013. "The Association between Dietary Patterns at Midlife and Health in Aging: An Observational Study." *Annals of Internal Medicine* 159, 9: 584–91.

Serra-Majem, Lluís, et al. 2006. "Scientific Evidence of Interventions Using the Mediterranean Diet: A Systematic Review." *Nutrition Reviews* 64, 2 (Pt 2): S27–47.

Schwingshackl, Lukas, et al. 2015. "Adherence to a Mediterranean Diet and Risk of Diabetes: A Systematic Review and Meta-analysis." *Public Health Nutrition* 18, 7: 1292–99.

Sofi, F., et al. 2014. "Mediterranean Diet and Health Status: An Updated Meta-analysis and a Proposal for a Literature-based Adherence Score." *Public Health Nutrition* 17: 2769–82.

Tosti, Valeria, et al. 2018. "Health Benefits of the Mediterranean Diet: Metabolic and Molecular Mechanisms." *Journals of Gerontology: Series A, Biological Sciences and Medical Sciences* 73, 3: 318–26.

Trichopoulou, A., et al. 2003. "Adherence to a Mediterranean Diet and Survival in a Greek Population." *New England Journal of Medicine* 348, 26: 2599–608.

Trichopoulou, A., et al. 1993. "The Macronutrient Composition of the Greek Diet: Estimates Derived from Six Case-Control Studies." *European Journal of Clinical Nutrition* 47, 8: 549–58.

Uusitupa, Matti, et al. 2019. "Prevention of Type 2 Diabetes by Lifestyle Changes: A Systematic Review and Meta-Analysis." *Nutrients* 11, 11: 2611.

Vujkovic, Marijana, et al. 2010. "The Preconception Mediterranean Dietary Pattern in Couples Undergoing in Vitro Fertilization/Intracytoplasmic Sperm Injection Treatment Increases the Chance of Pregnancy." *Fertility and Sterility* 94, 6: 2096–101.

World Cancer Research Fund International. 2018. *Diet, Nutrition, Physical Activity and Cancer: A Global Perspective—The Third Expert Report.* London, UK: World Cancer Research Fund International. Available from: https://www.wcrf.org/dietandcancer

Acknowledgments

This book has existed in my mind and in my heart for as long as I can remember. I am forever grateful for the village that helped me turn this vision into the beautiful book you are holding in your hands today. This book was written in isolation during the COVID-19 pandemic, newborn in tow. Writing about food culture and creating recipes meant for sharing, whilst siloed in our homes, gave me (and all of you, I'm sure) new meaning to the family table. If the pandemic taught us anything, it's that life is lived in the moments, and that many of these moments happen in the kitchen. So thank you for your support and for bringing this book into your home—may it create memorable times for you and your family.

A very special thank you to my family. You are the soul of this book. Thank you to my nonni, for the memories you created around the table that inspired the recipes in this book. I miss you. To my parents, Domenico and Nella, this book literally could not have been written if it weren't for you. Thank you for exemplifying such positive food culture in our home—I now realize what a gift that was and how difficult it must have been to make all those meals from scratch while working so hard. I value it so much. Thank you to my sister, Claudia, for being my number one fan and championing my work, rain or shine. You have inspired me to keep going after my dreams more times than you know. Thank you to my husband, Cosimo, for your love and your unwavering belief in me. I feel so lucky to have you by my side and to share my meals with you every day.

Thank you to Ariel Tarr, for your passion and attention to detail, which shines through in every photo. Thank you to Michael Linnington—your styling brings recipes to life on the page. Thank you to Annie Lachapelle

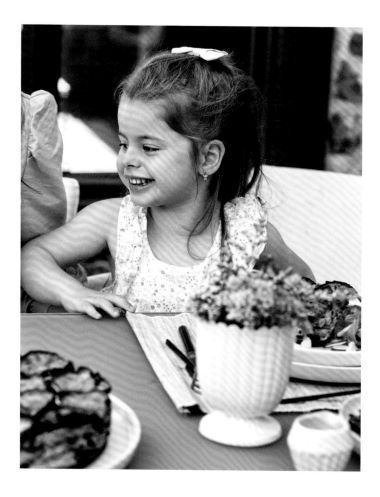

for your vision and to Carolina for your energy and help in the kitchen. You all made the photoshoot an absolute dream of an experience.

A special thank you to my wonderful editor, Rachel Brown, for your faith in me and in this project, since day one. Thank you for believing in my vision, for working so hard to honor it, and for making this book better than I ever thought it could be. I am forever grateful for you.

Thank you to Robert McCullough for your trust and support, which have allowed me to realize this dream project.

Thank you to Lisa Jager, for designing such a beautiful book. To Judith, Lana, Whitney, Michelle, Charlotte, and the entire Appetite team—thank you for your precious work. It is an honor to be part of the Appetite family and to work alongside you all to bring this book into people's homes.

Index